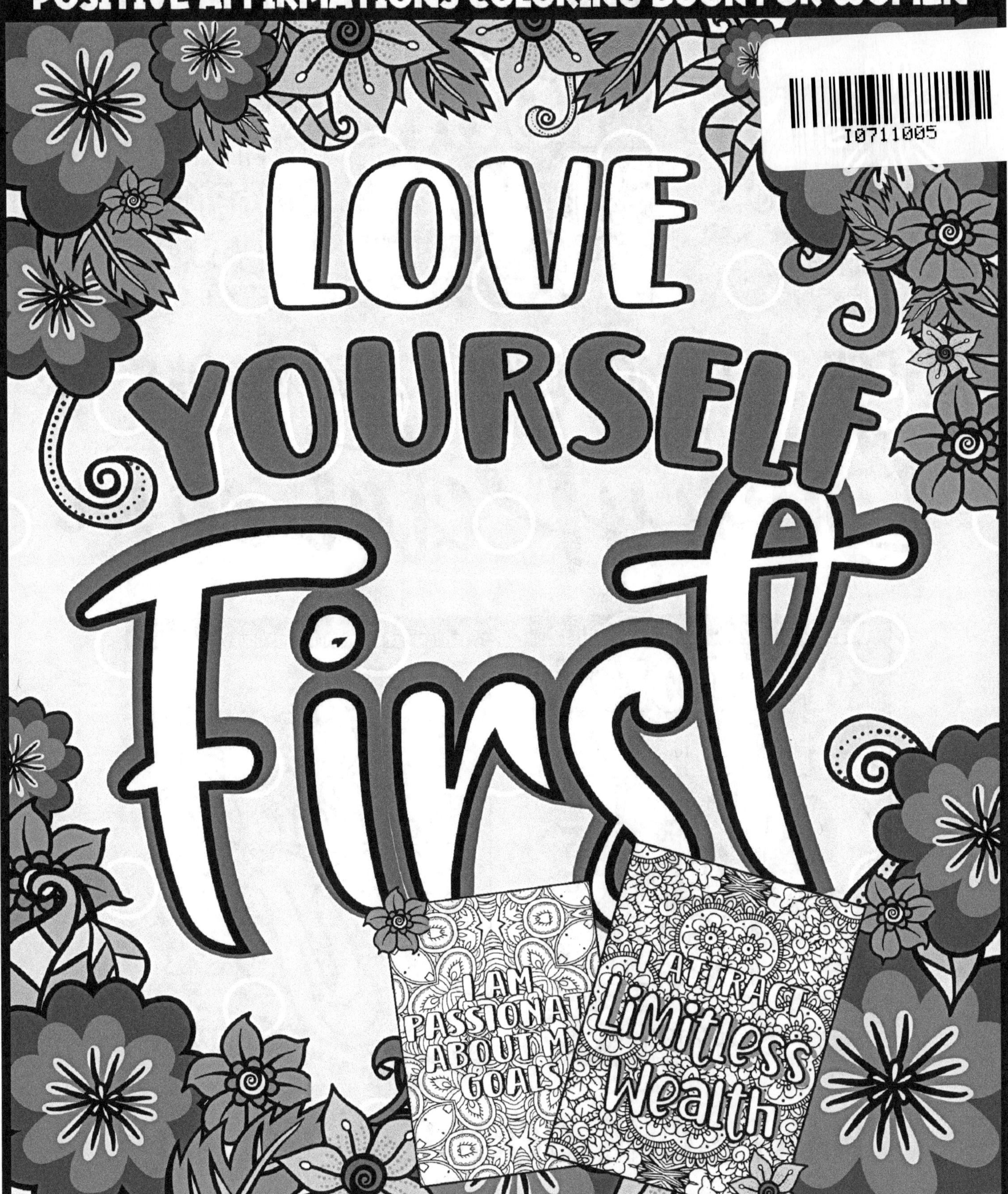

POSITIVE AFFIRMATIONS COLORING BOOK FOR WOMEN
LOVE YOURSELF First
I AM PASSIONAT ABOUT M GOALS
I ATTRACT Limitless Wealth

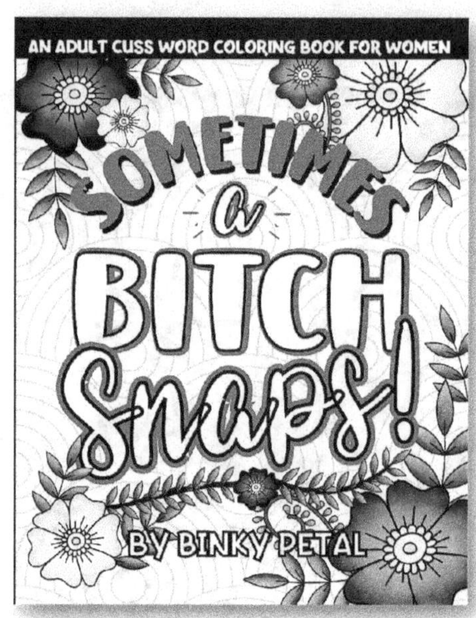

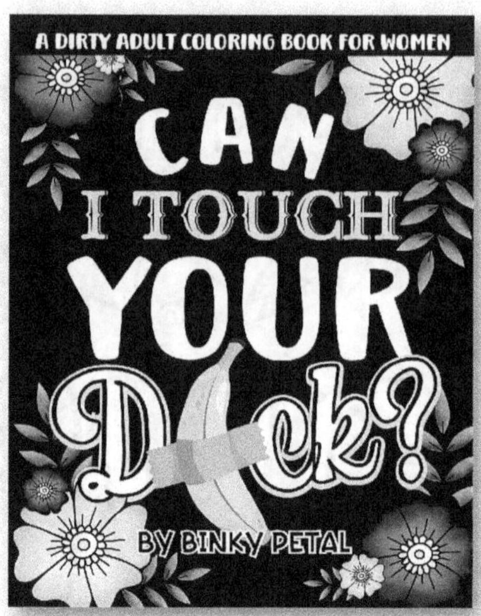

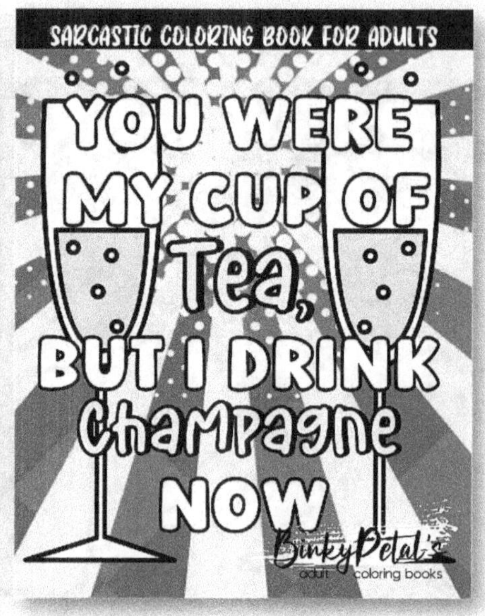

CHECK OUT MORE OF OUR BOOKS AT:

BinkyPetal.com

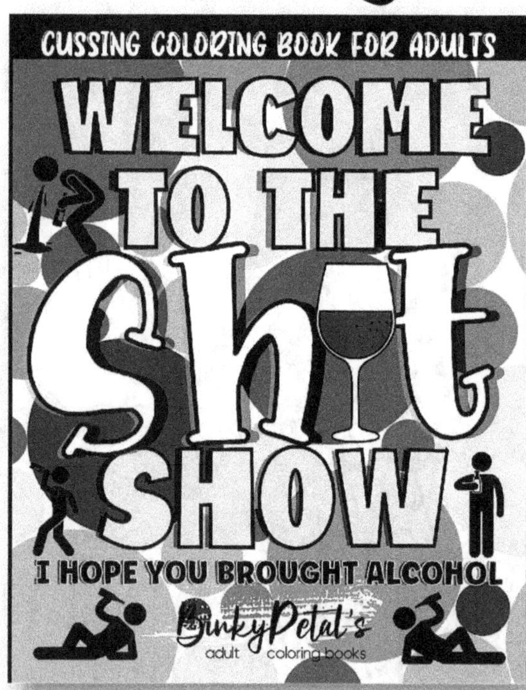

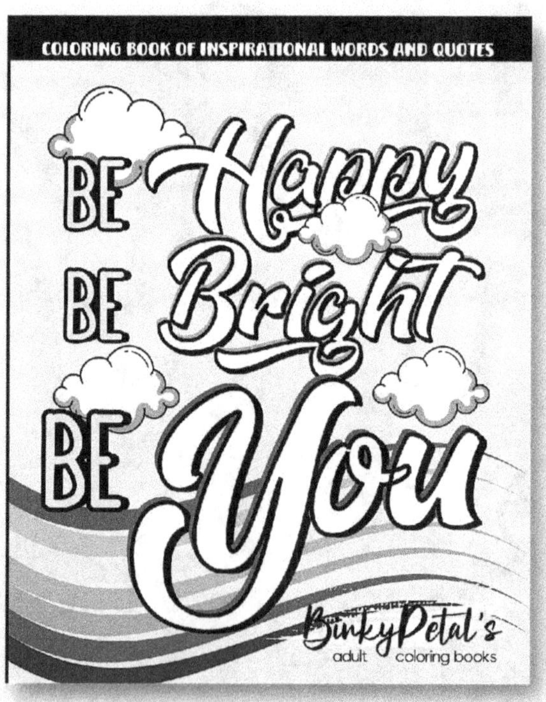

WANT SOME GOODIES? GO TO:

BINKYPETALDIGITAL.COM

A LITTLE SAMPLE

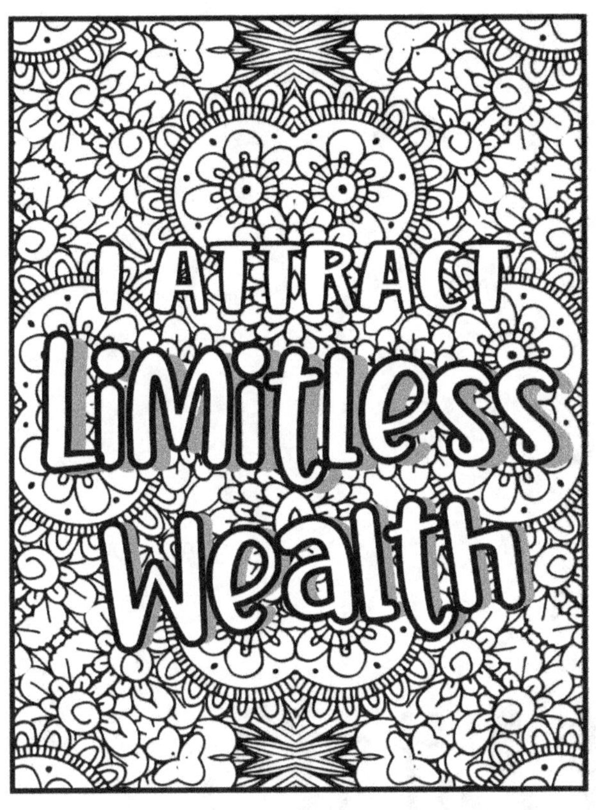

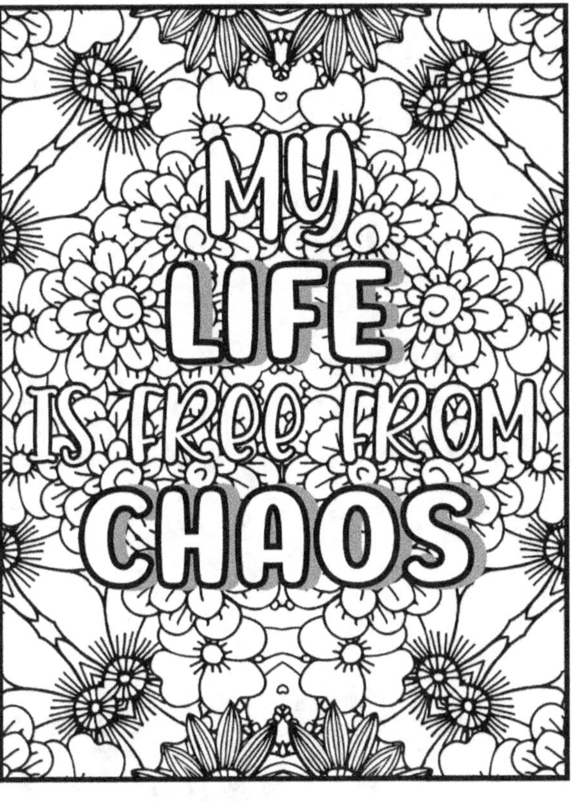

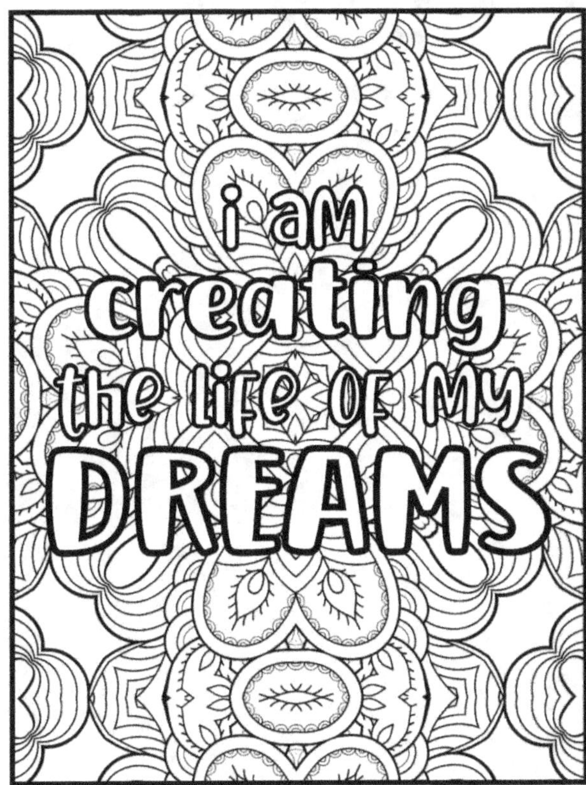

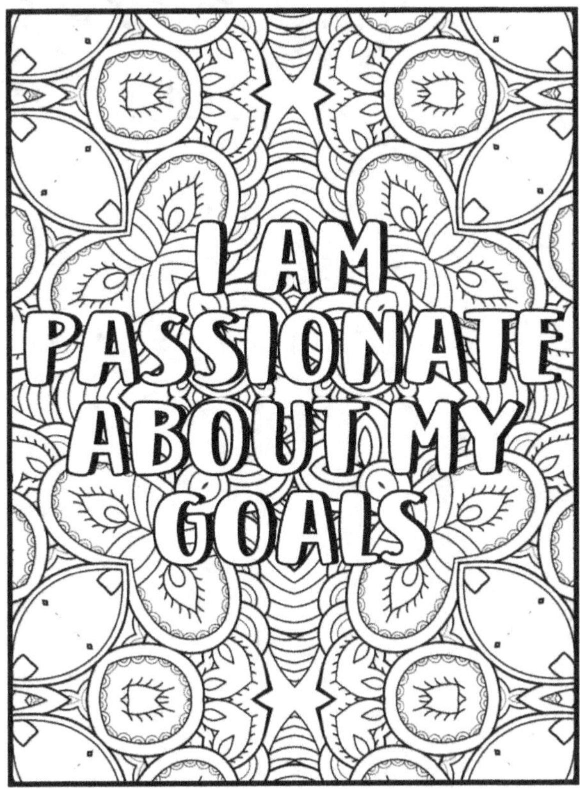

BinkyPetal's

adult   coloring books

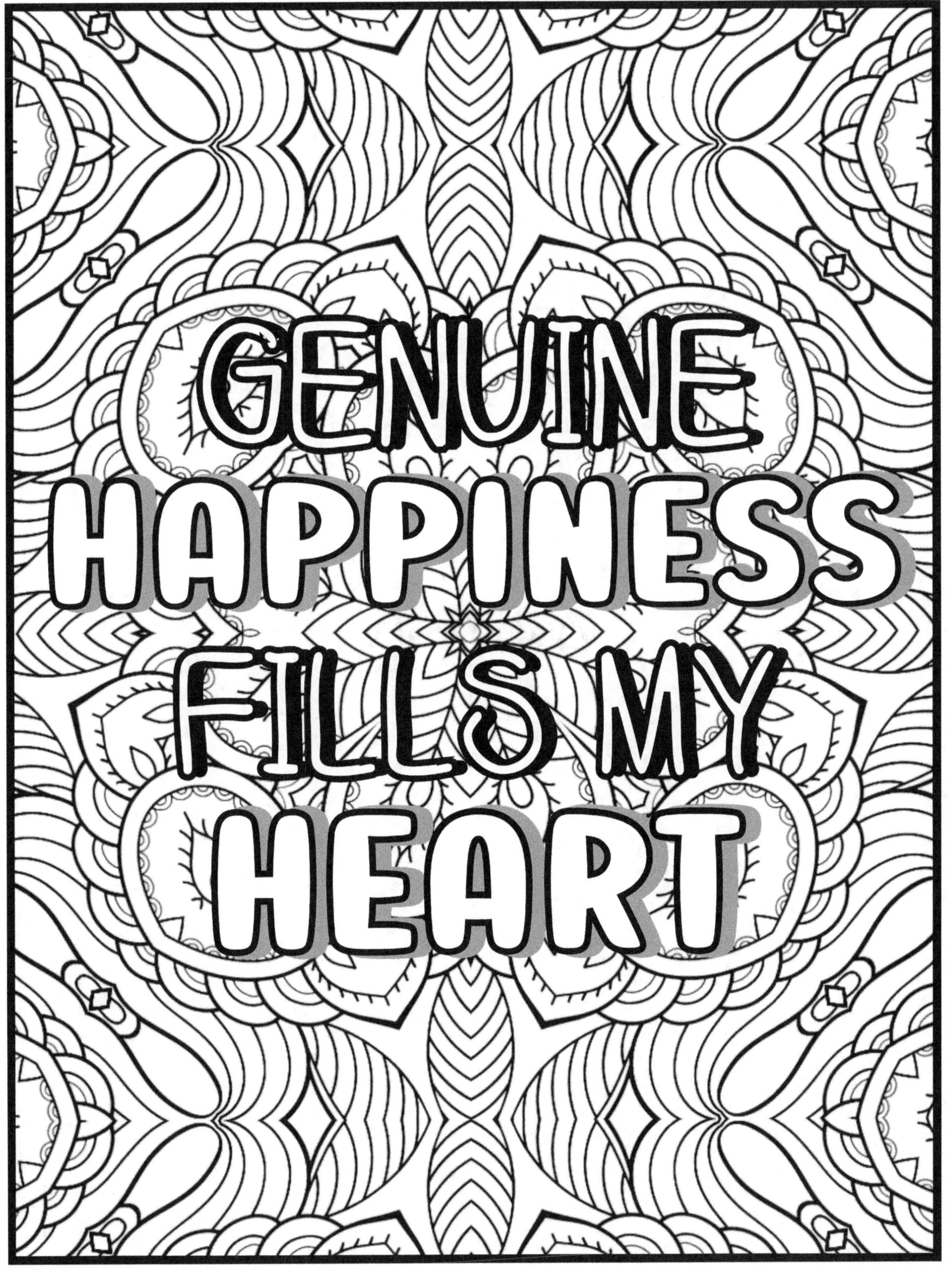

GENUINE HAPPINESS FILLS MY HEART

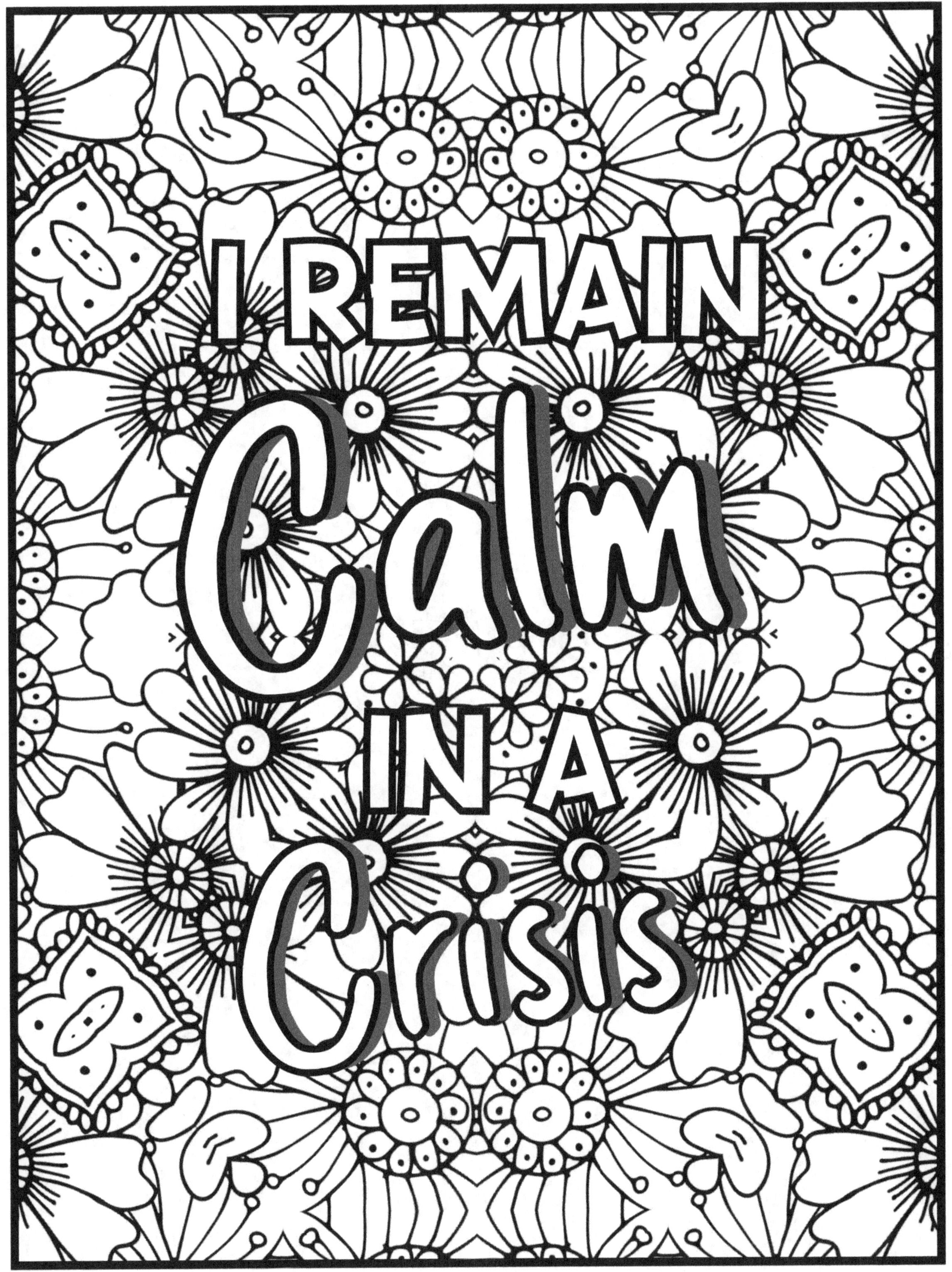

I REMAIN
Calm
IN A
Crisis

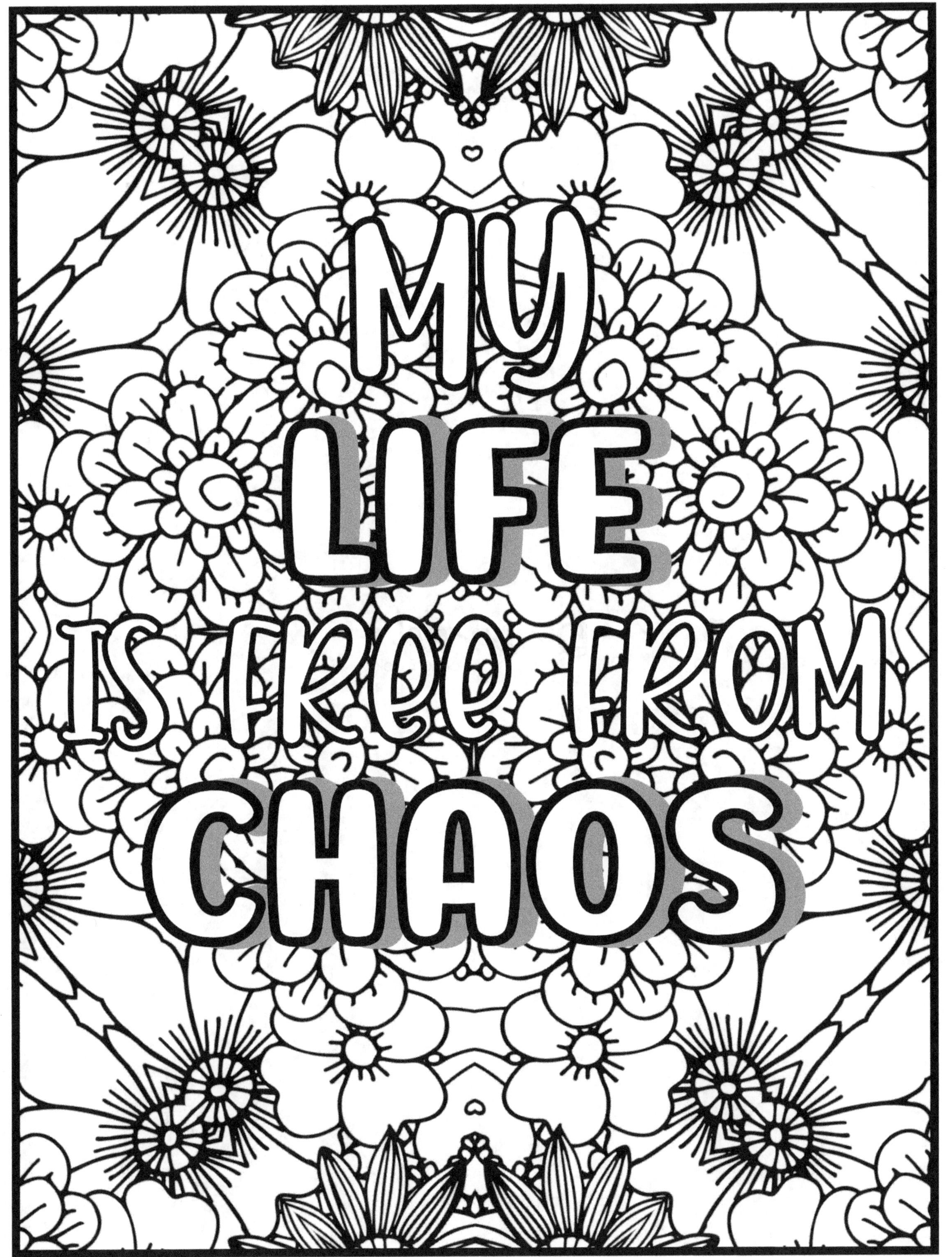

MY
LIFE
IS FREE FROM
CHAOS

BinkyPetal's
adult coloring books

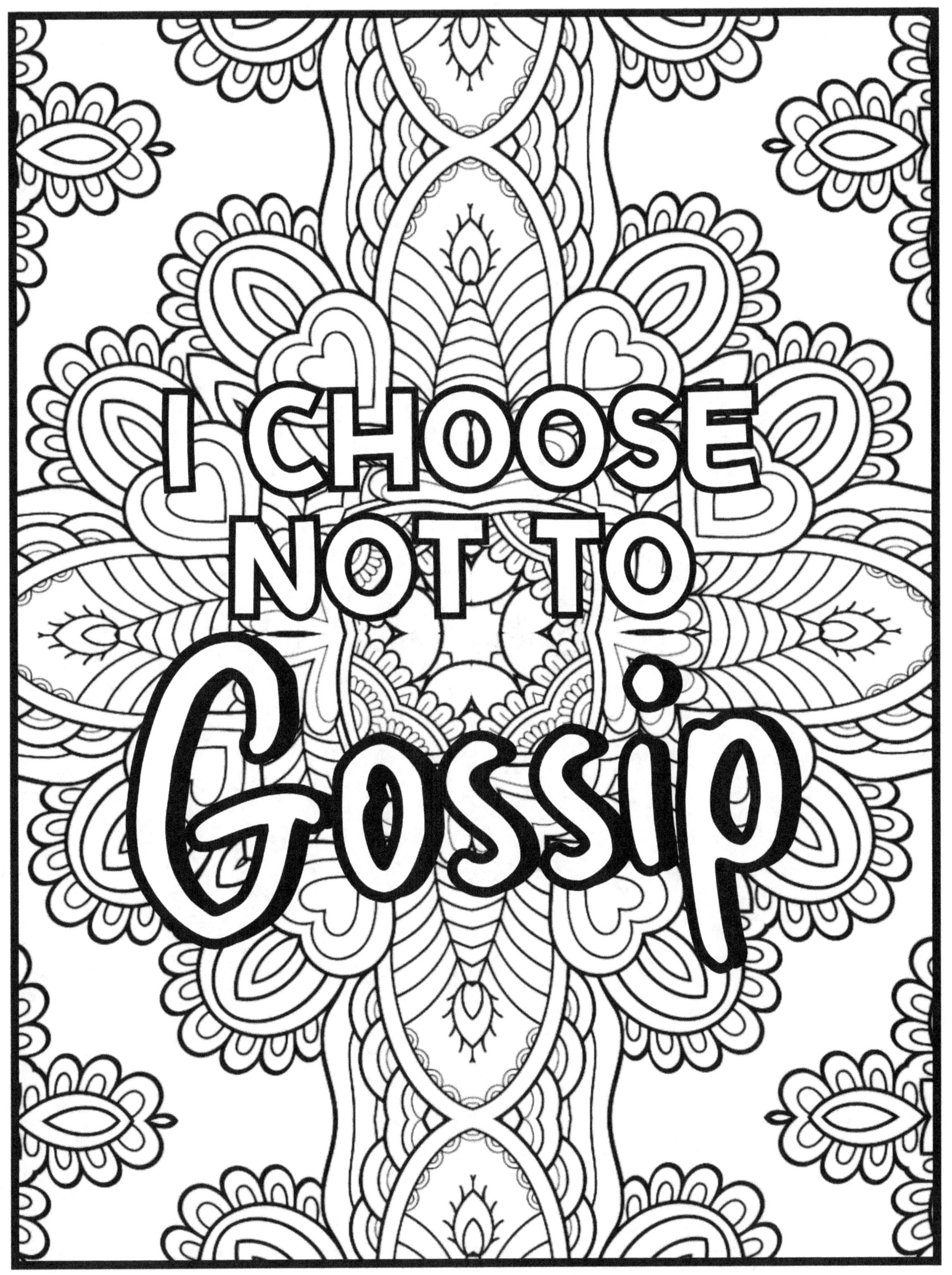
I CHOOSE
NOT TO
Gossip

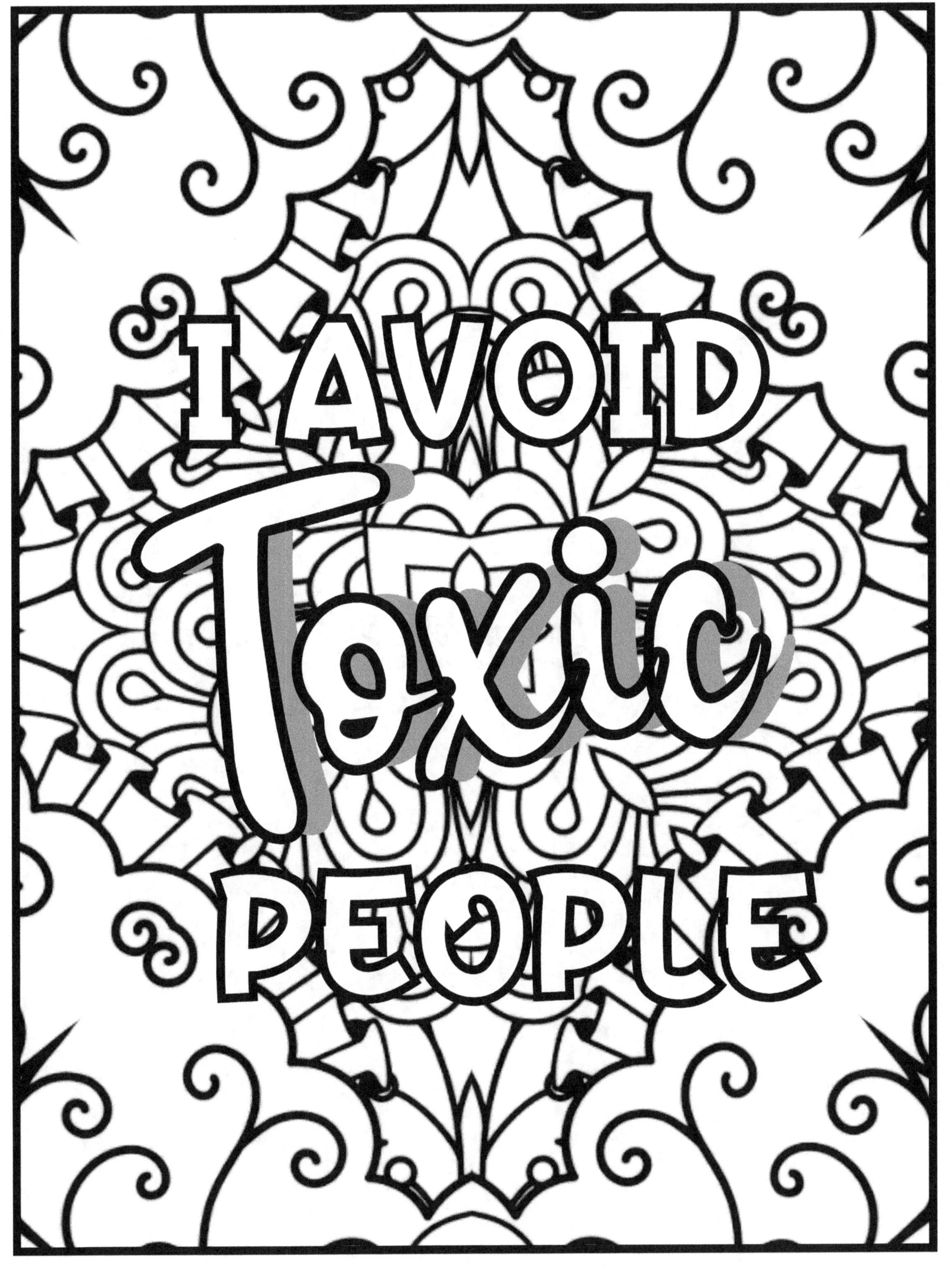

I AVOID
Toxic
PEOPLE

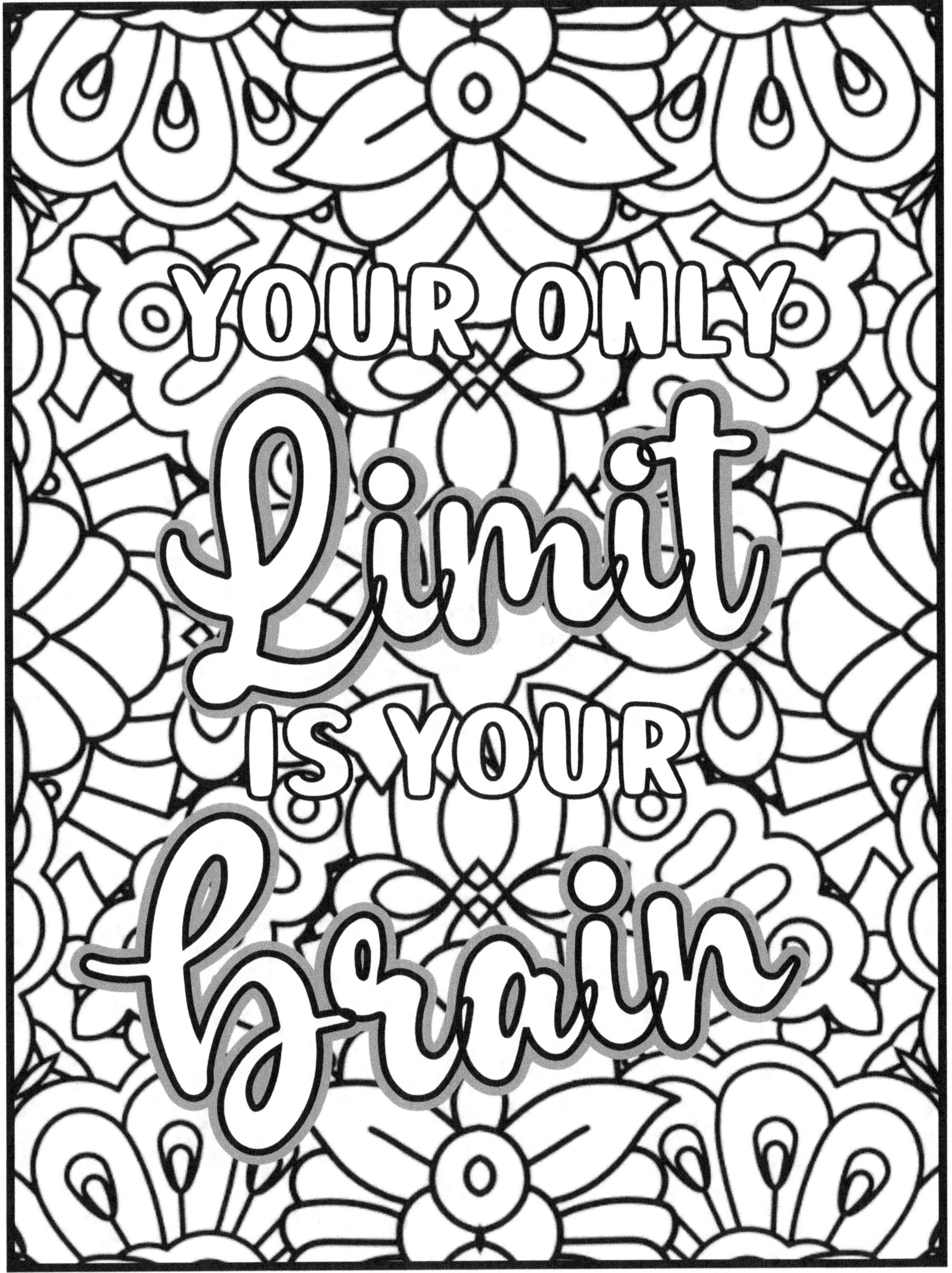

YOUR ONLY
Limit
IS YOUR
brain

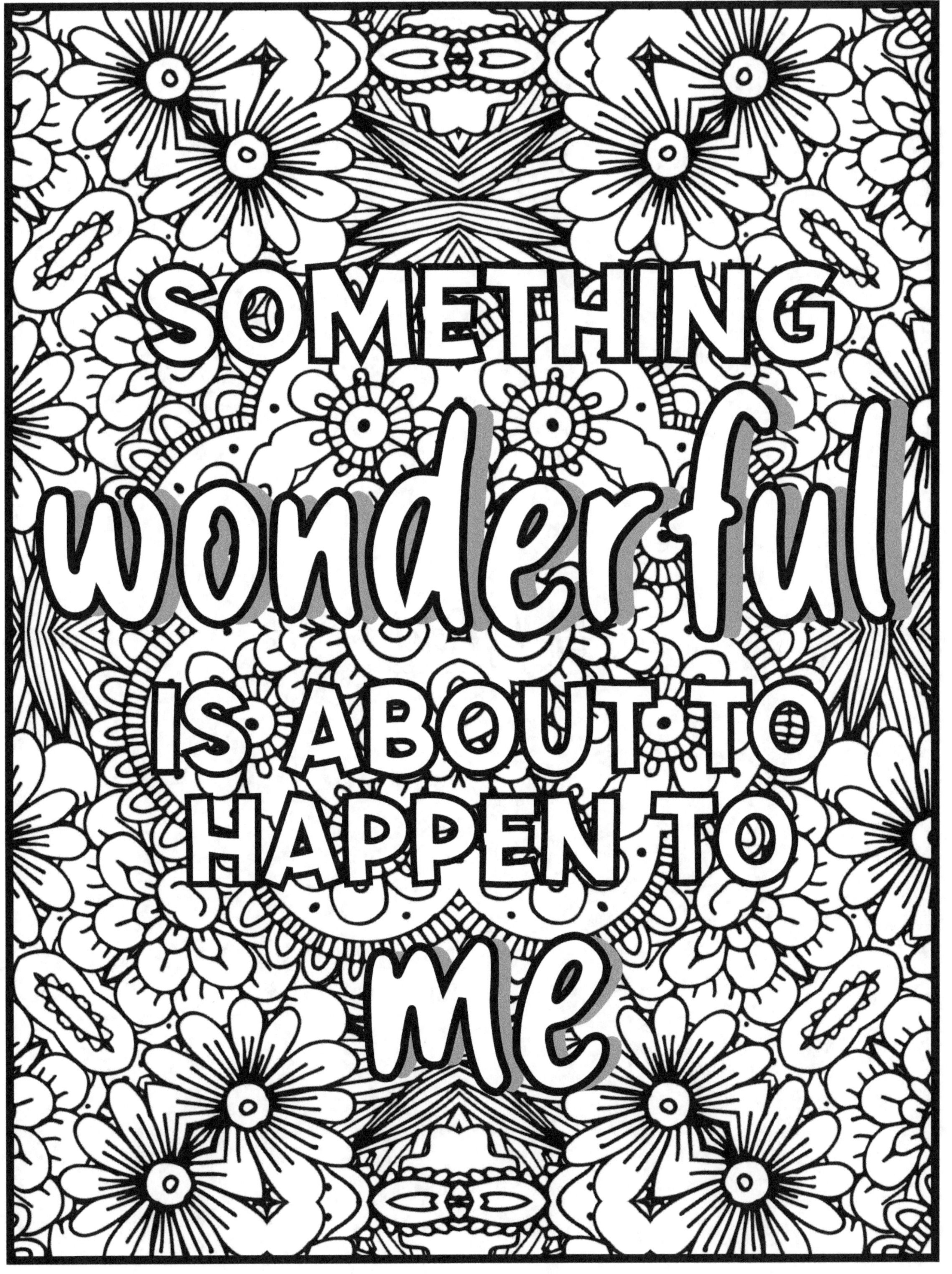

SOMETHING
wonderful
IS ABOUT TO
HAPPEN TO
ME

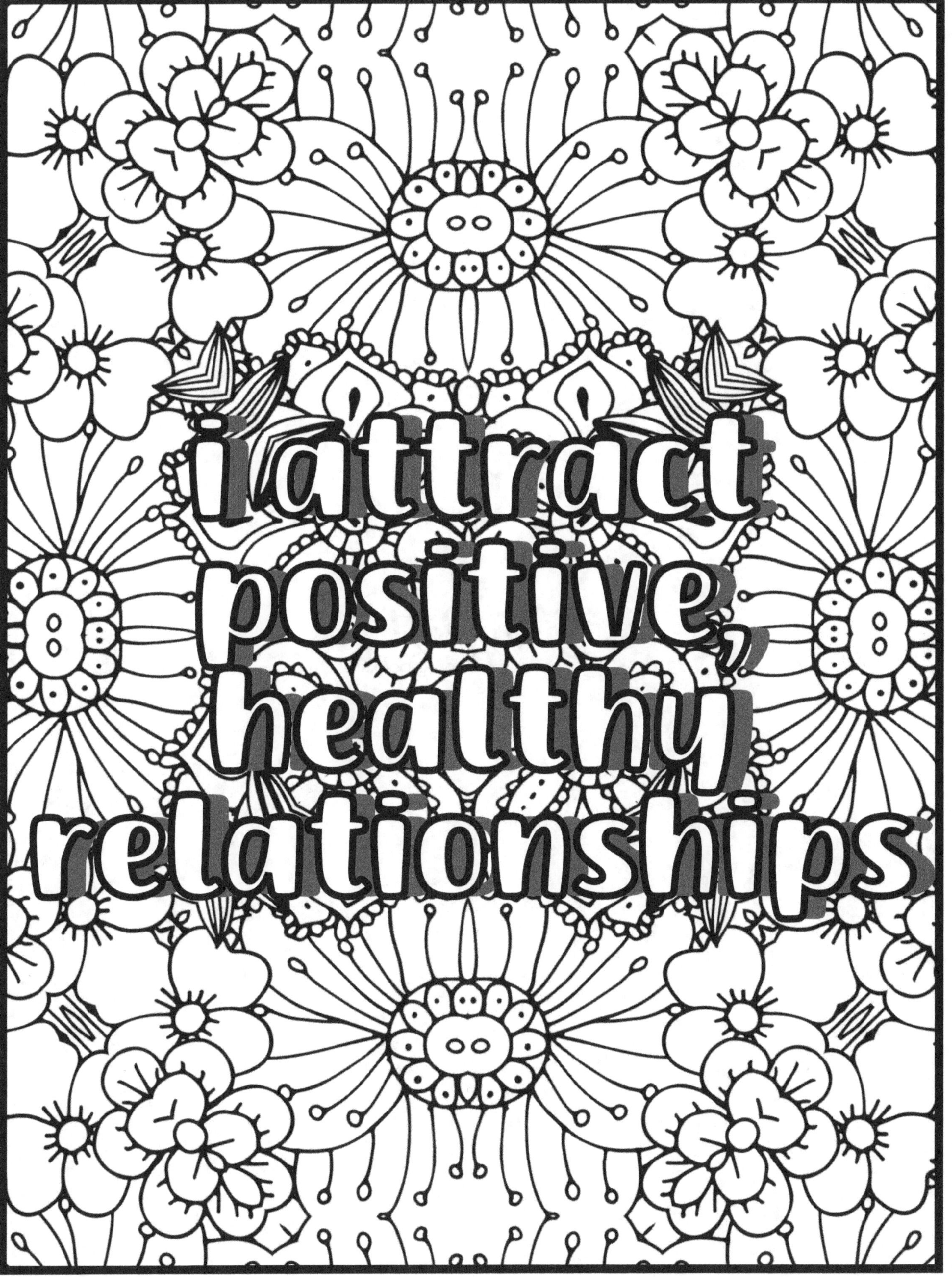
i attract
positive,
healthy
relationships

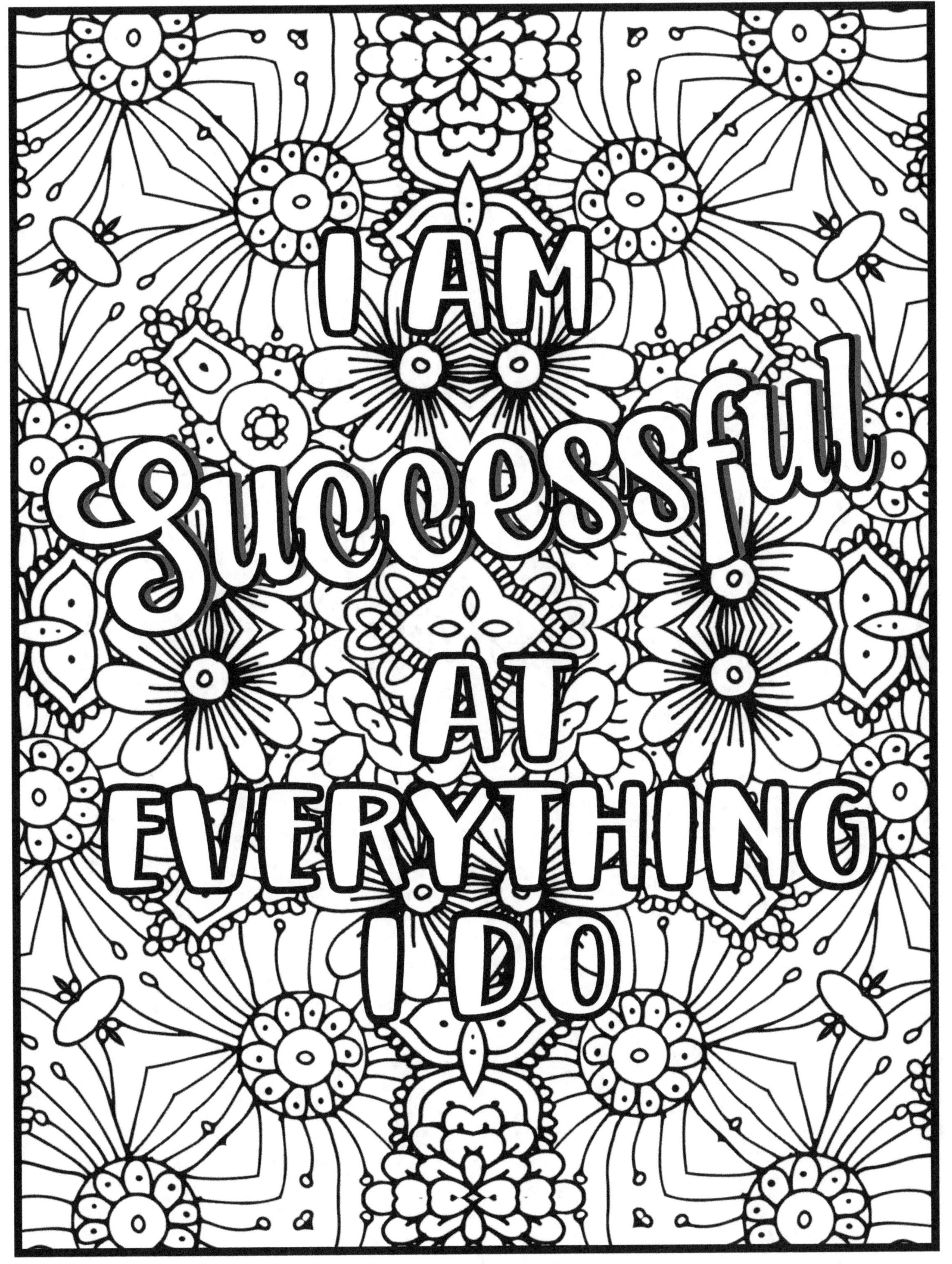

I AM
Successful
AT
EVERYTHING
I DO

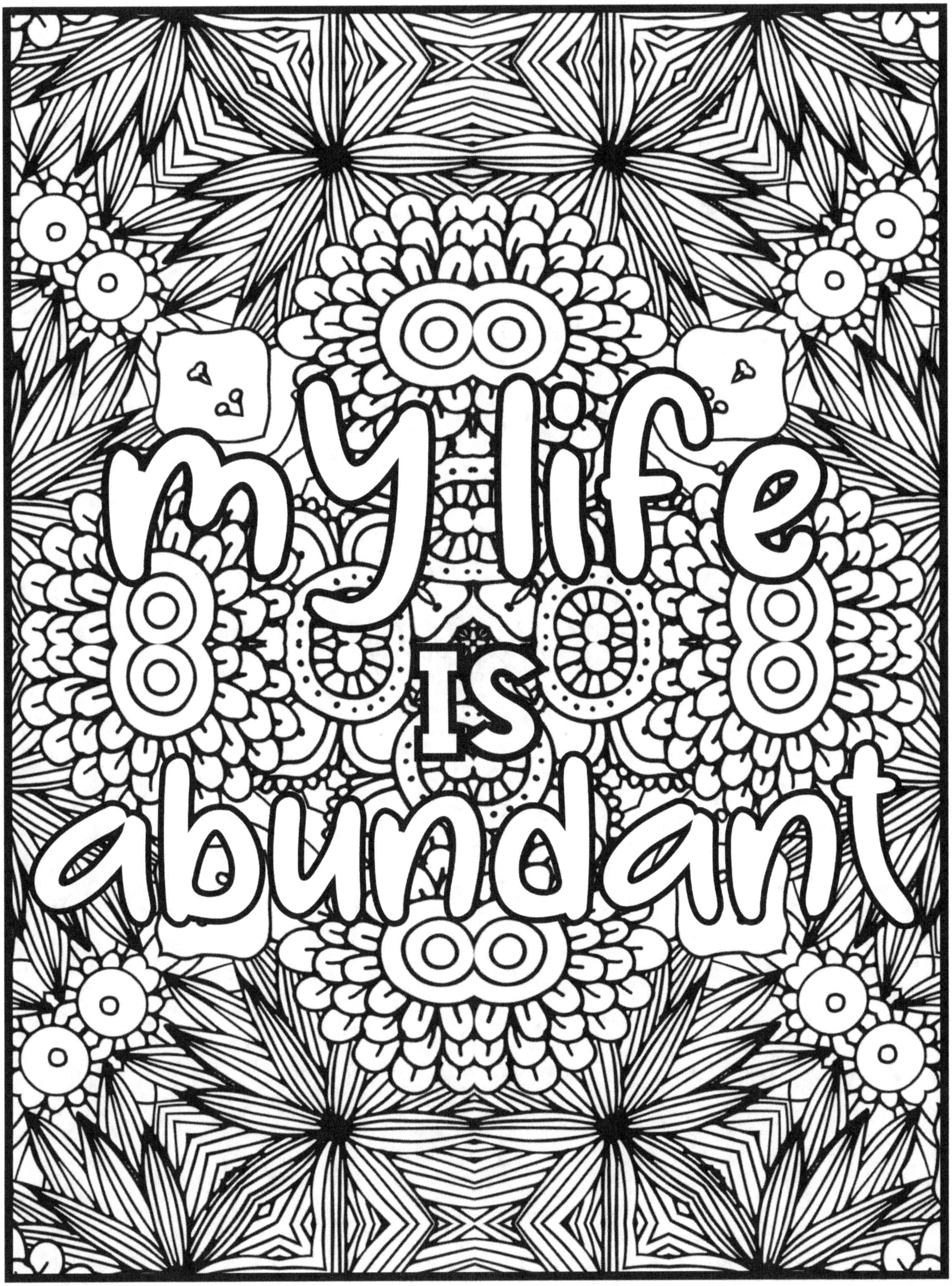
my life is abundant

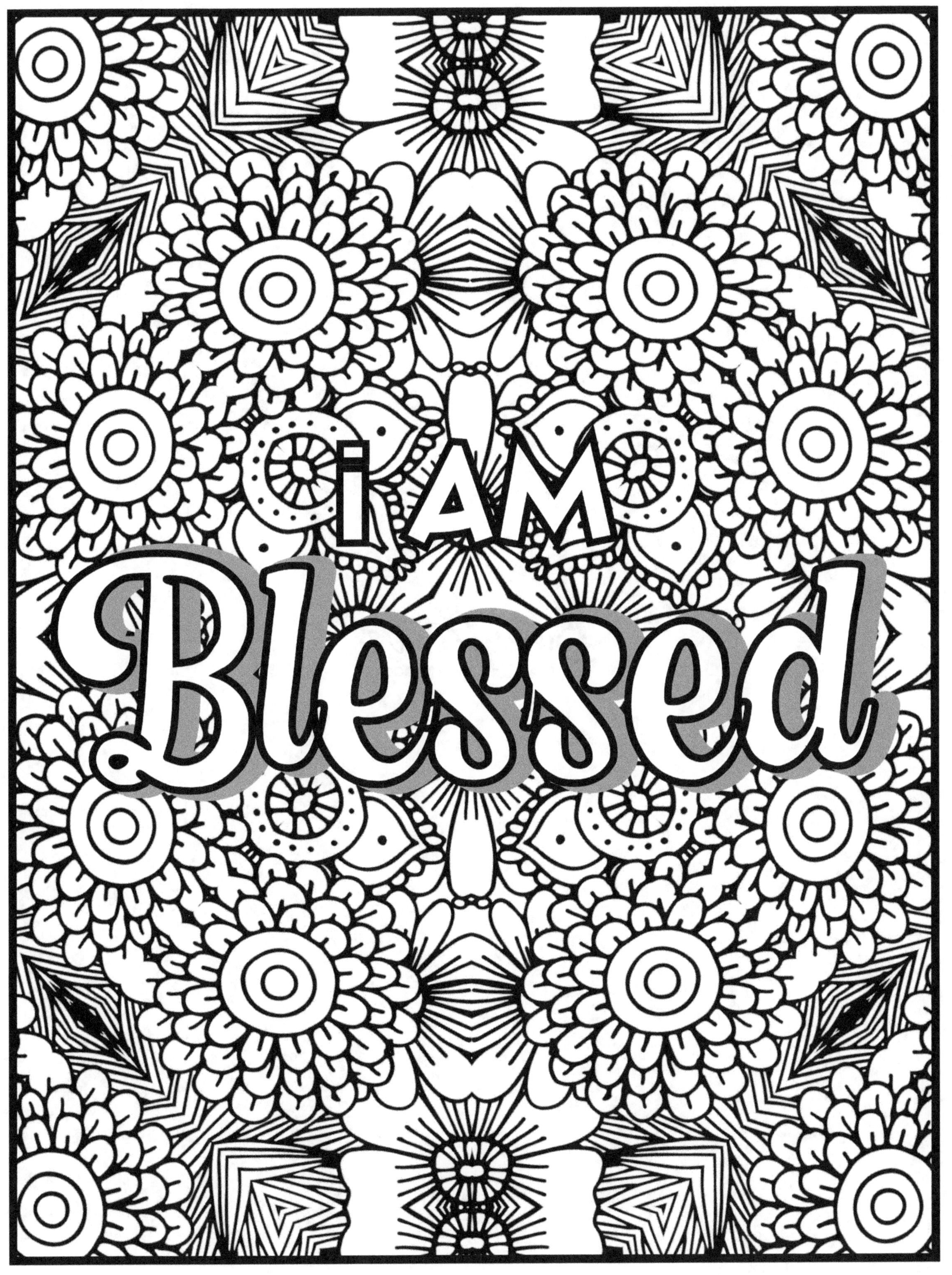

i AM
Blessed

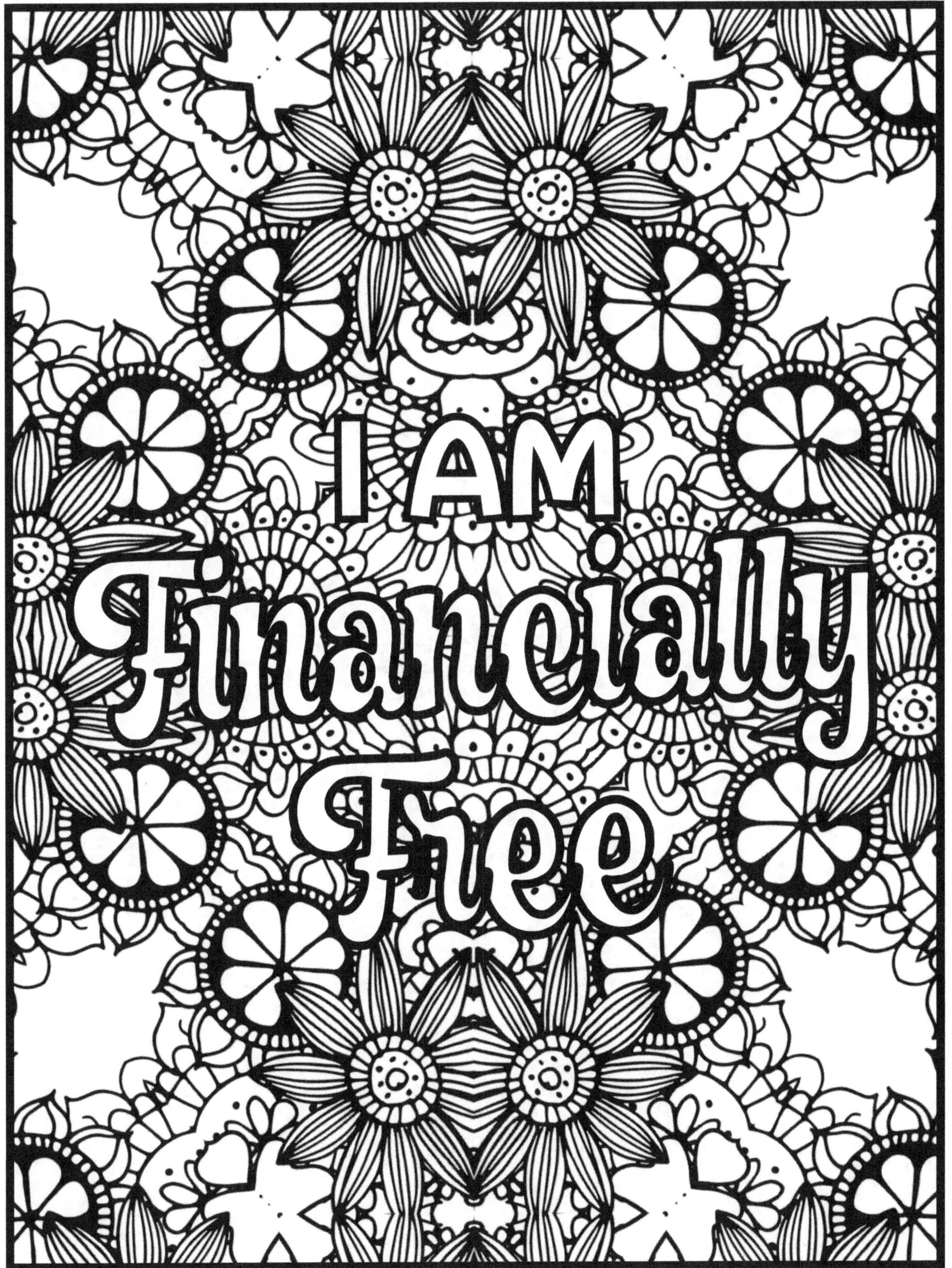

I AM
Financially
Free

BinkyPetal's
adult coloring books

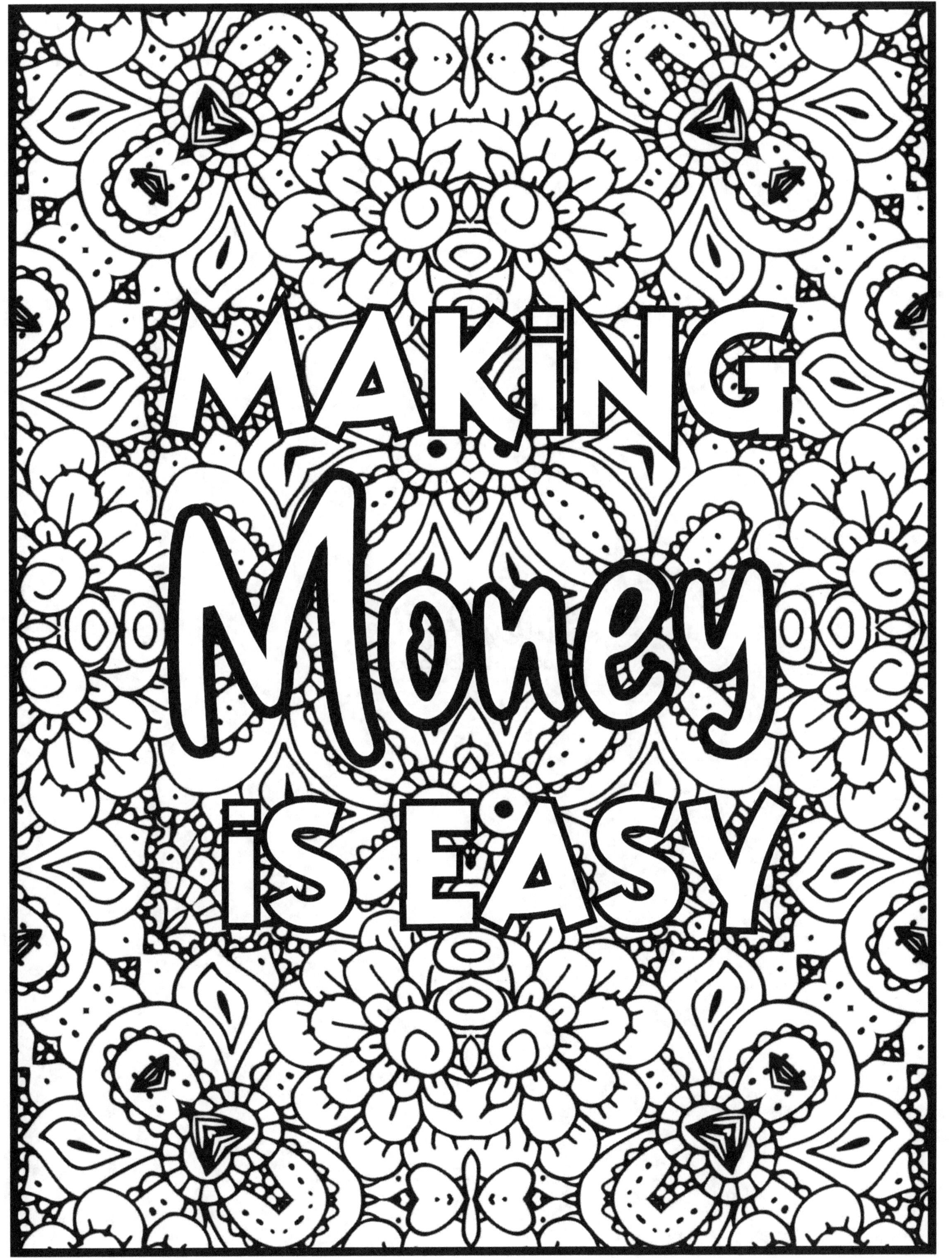

MAKING
Money
IS EASY

BinkyPetal's
adult coloring books

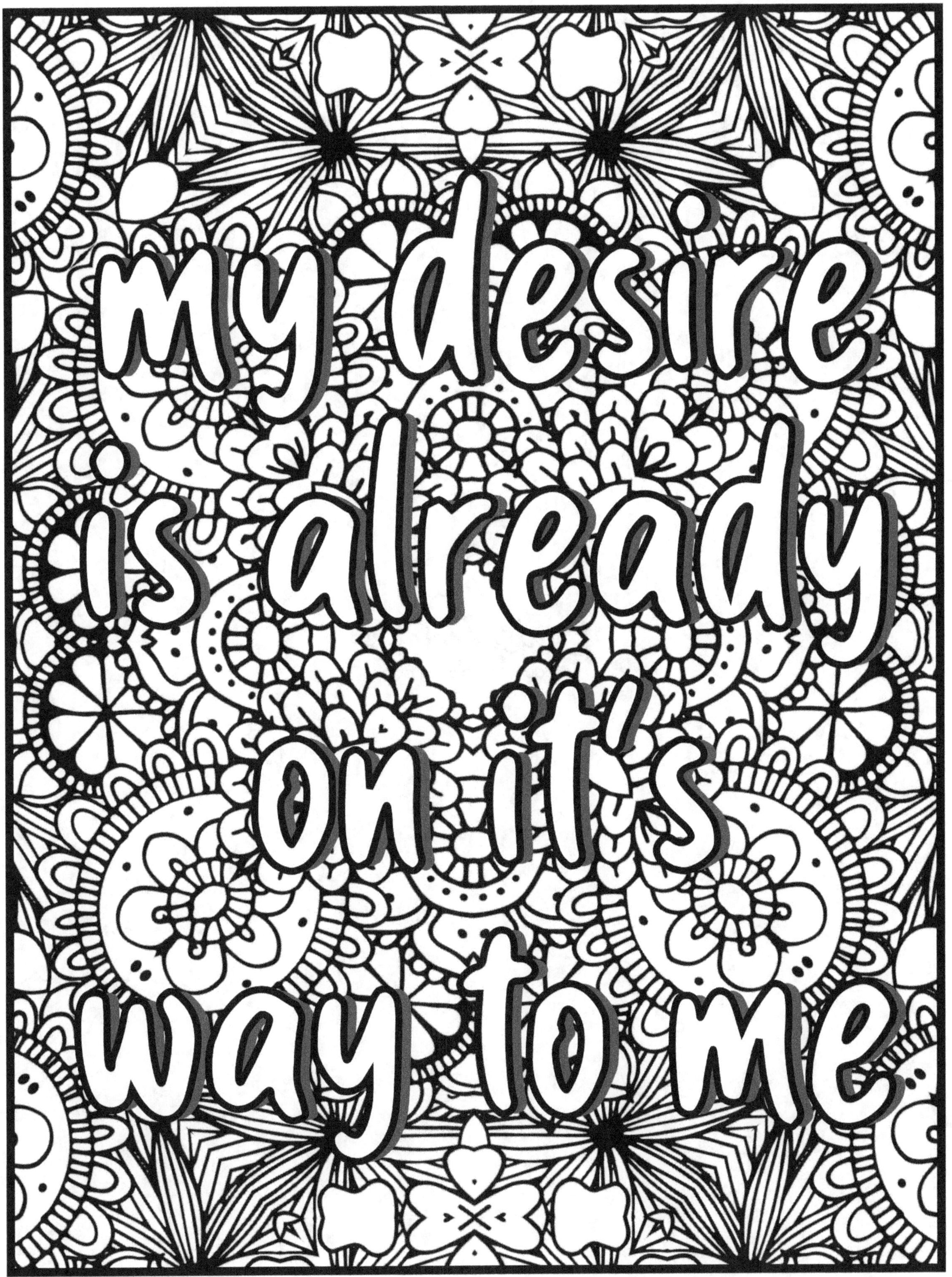

My desire
is already
on it's
way to me

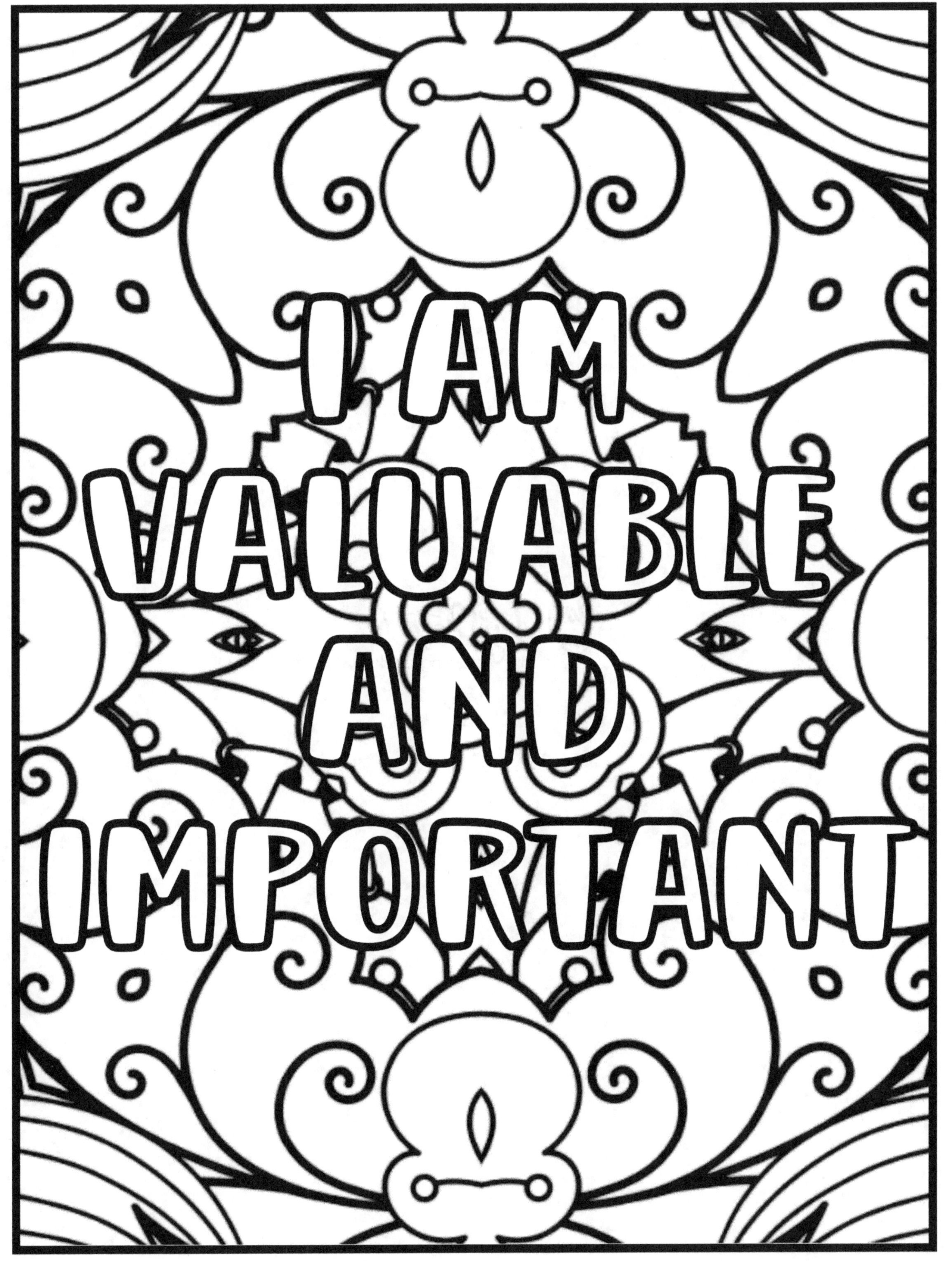

I AM
VALUABLE
AND
IMPORTANT

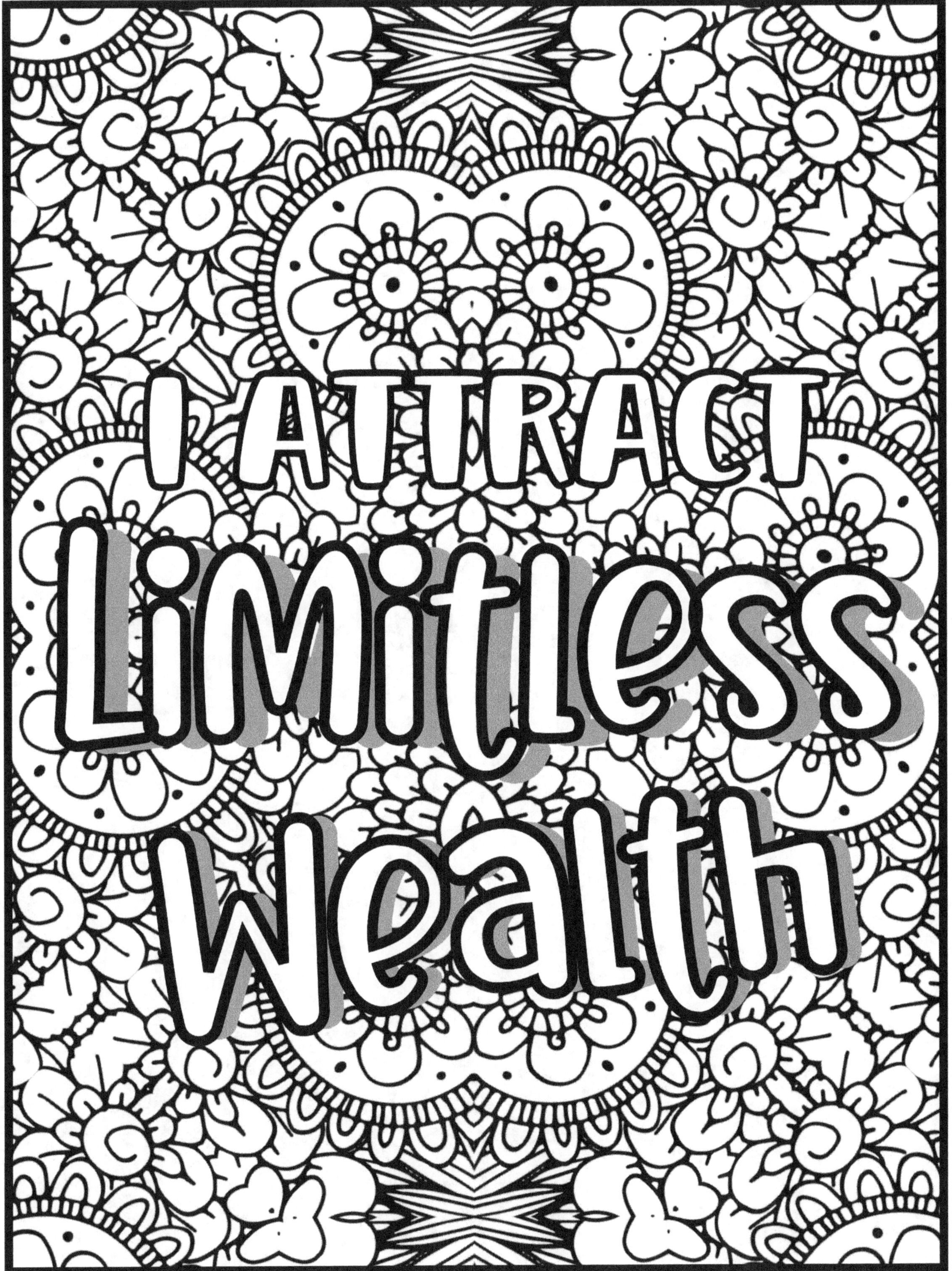

I ATTRACT
Limitless
Wealth

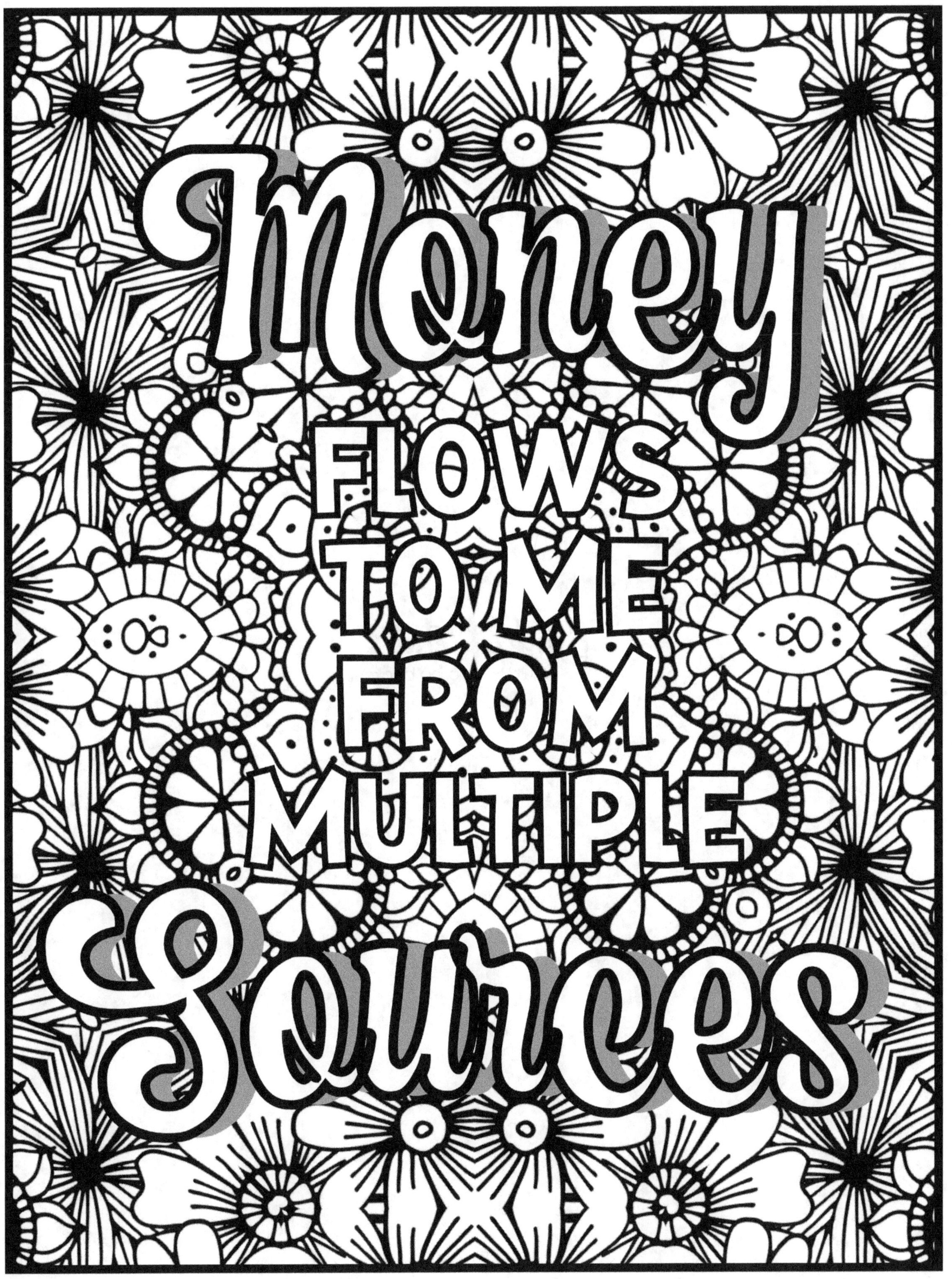

Money
FLOWS
TO ME
FROM
MULTIPLE
Sources

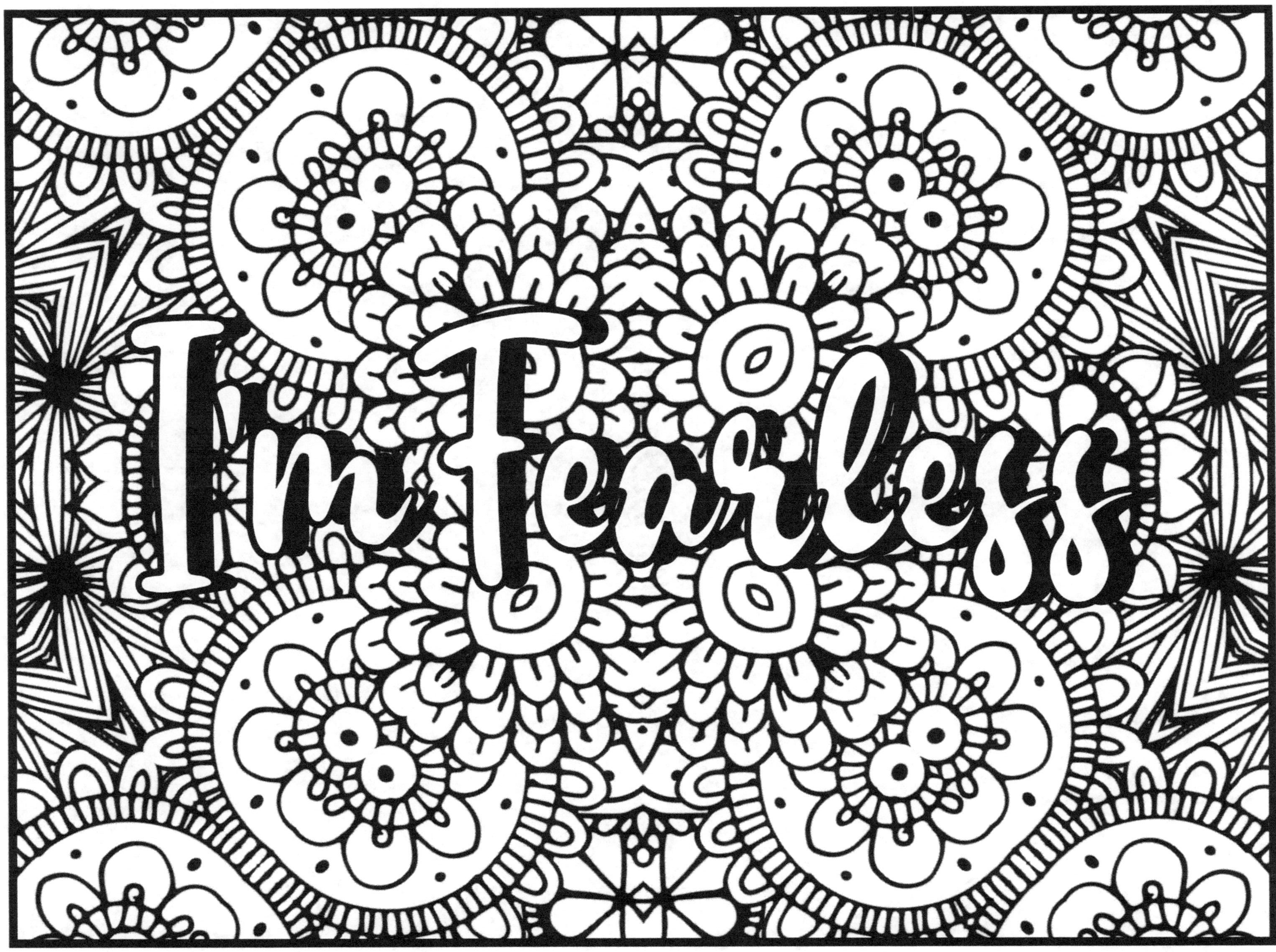
I'm Fearless

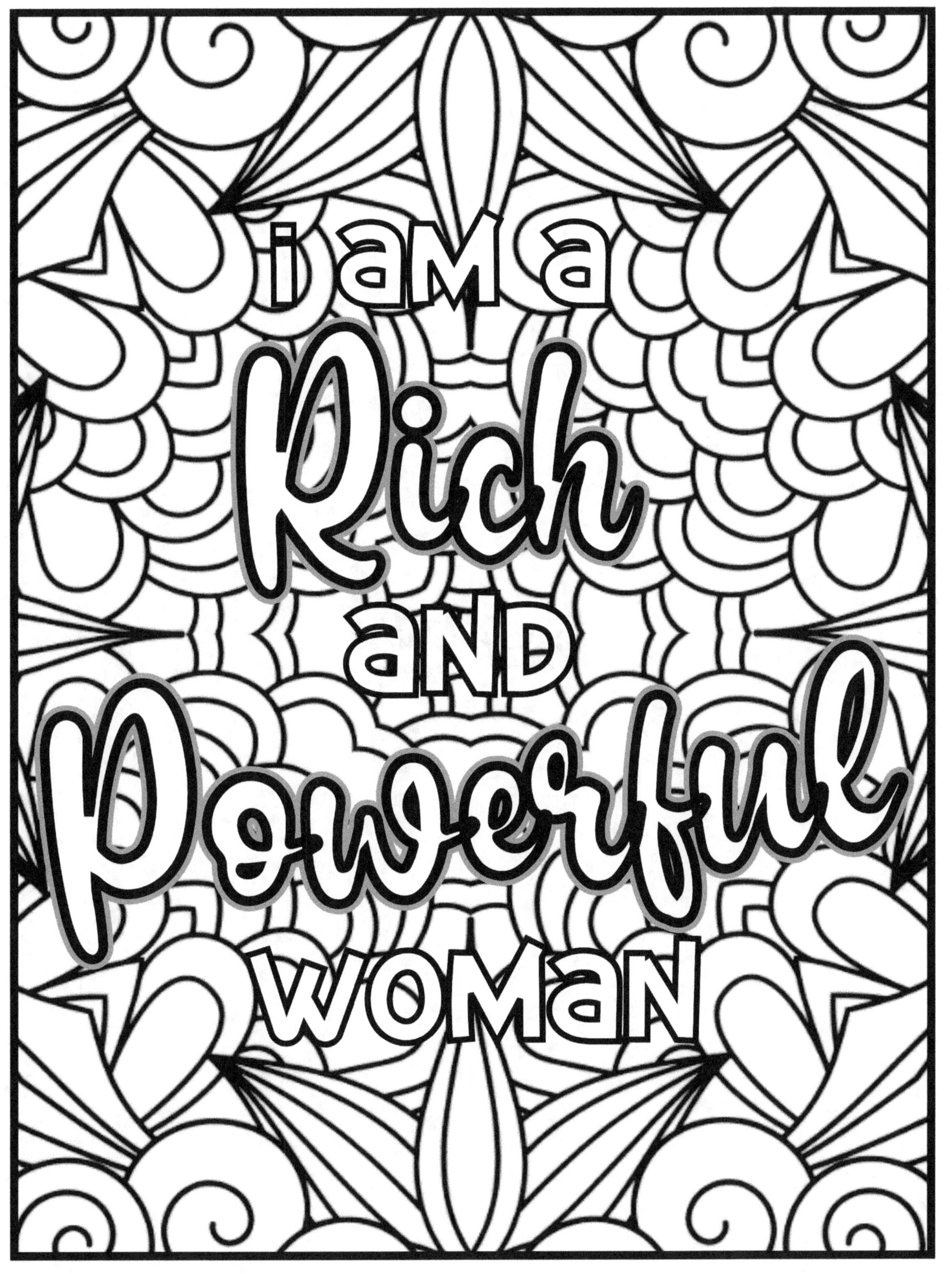

i am a
Rich
and
Powerful
woman

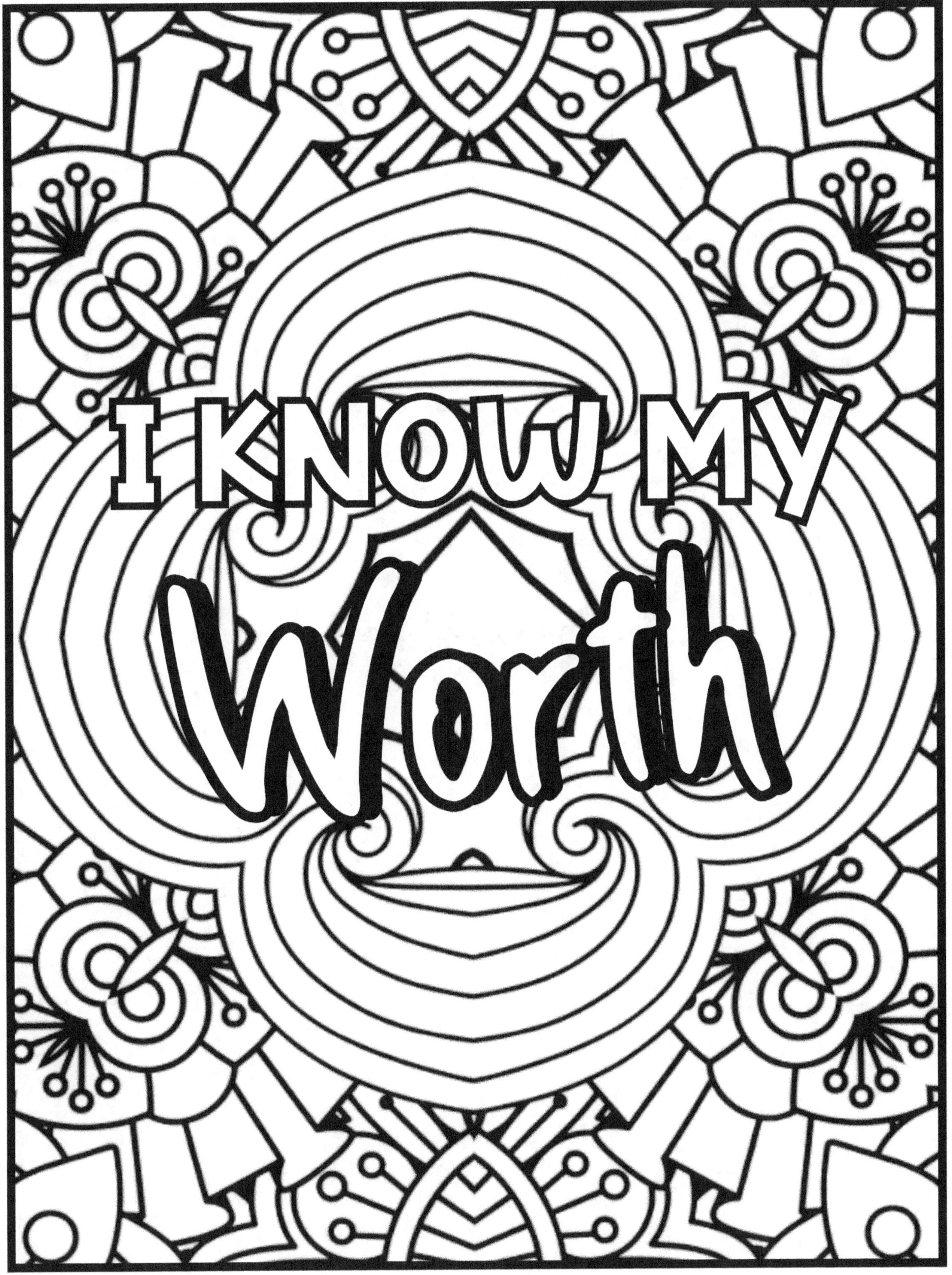

I KNOW MY
Worth

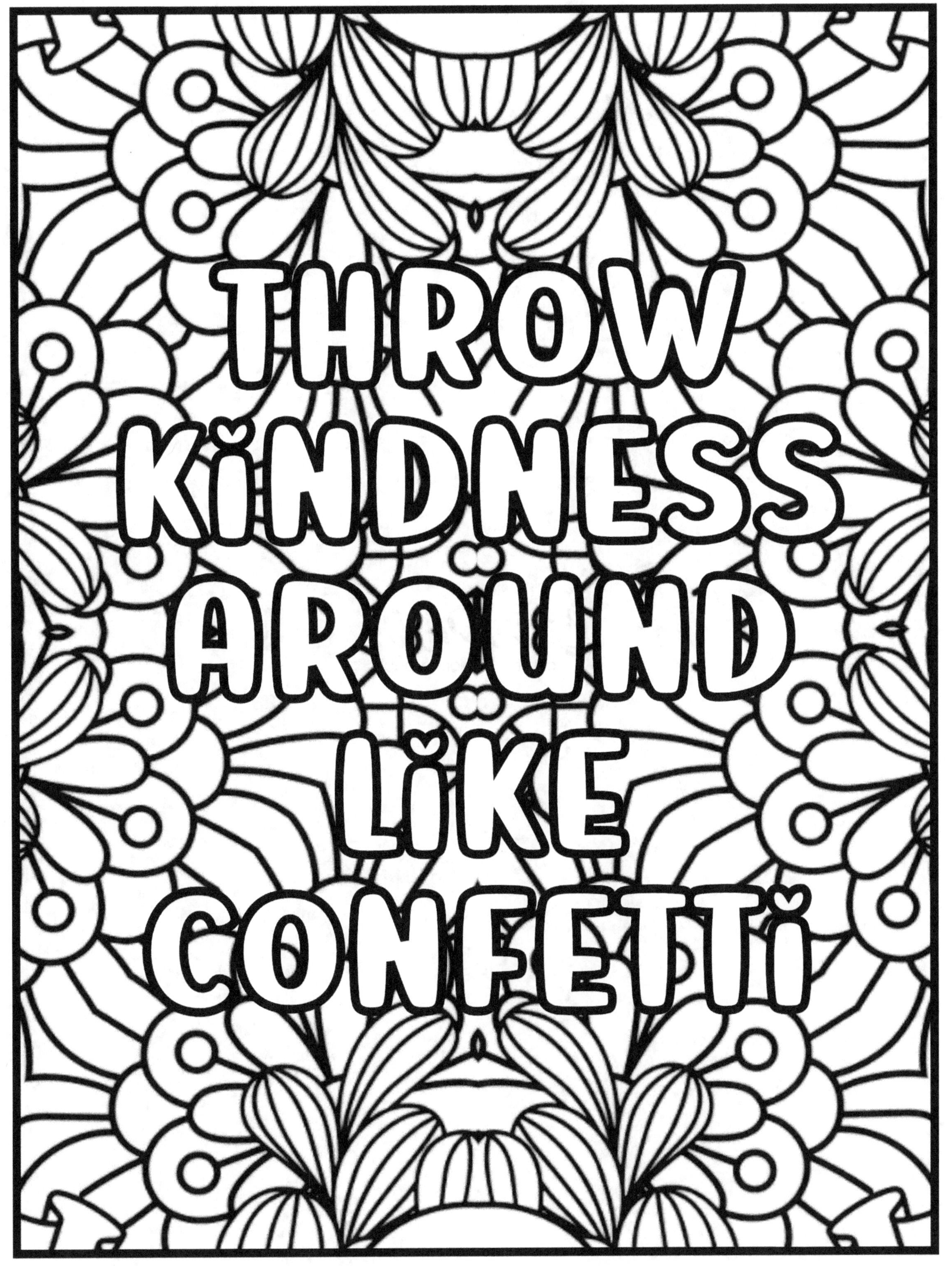
THROW
KINDNESS
AROUND
LIKE
CONFETTI

BinkyPetal's
adult coloring books

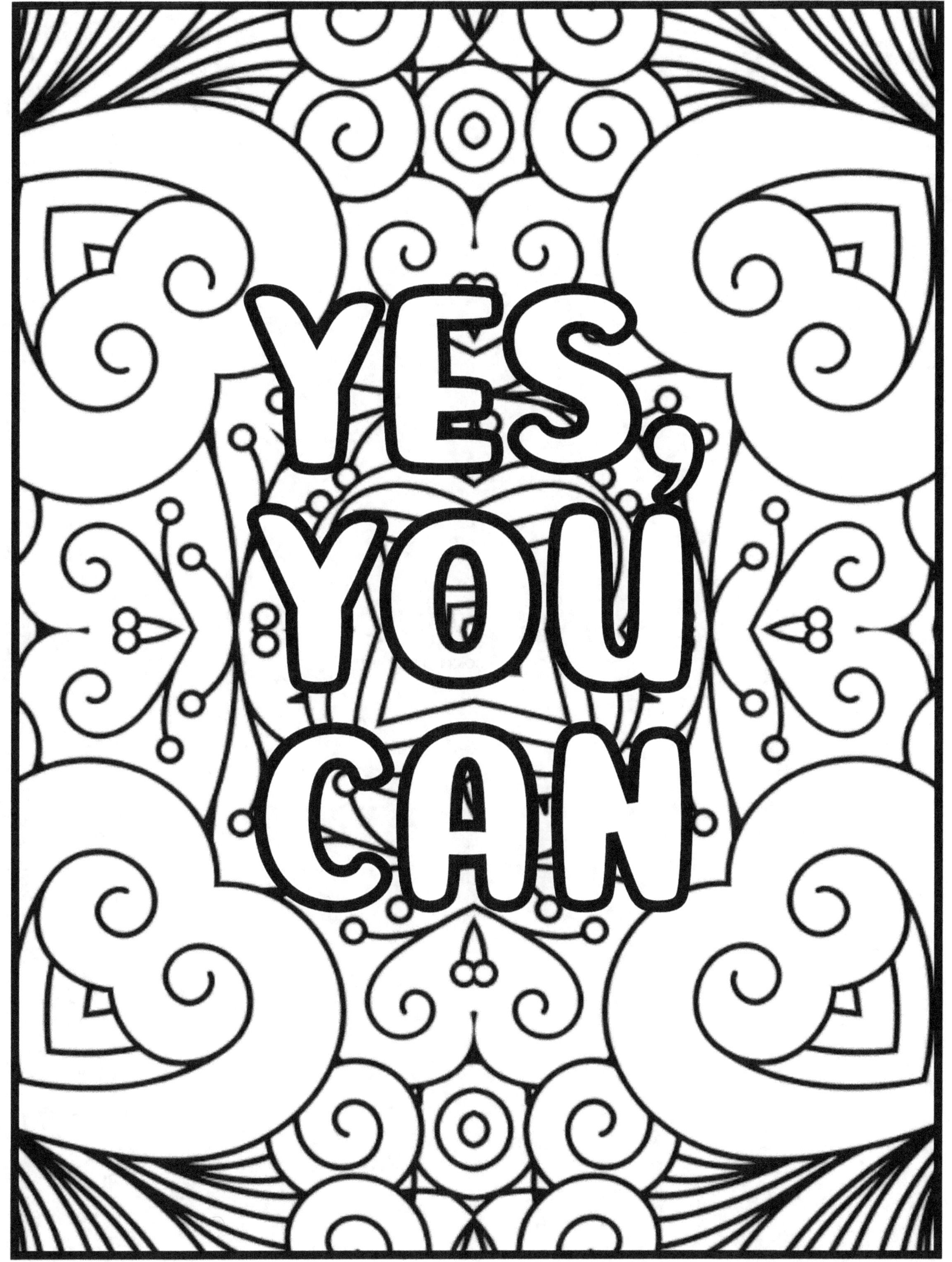
YES,
YOU
CAN

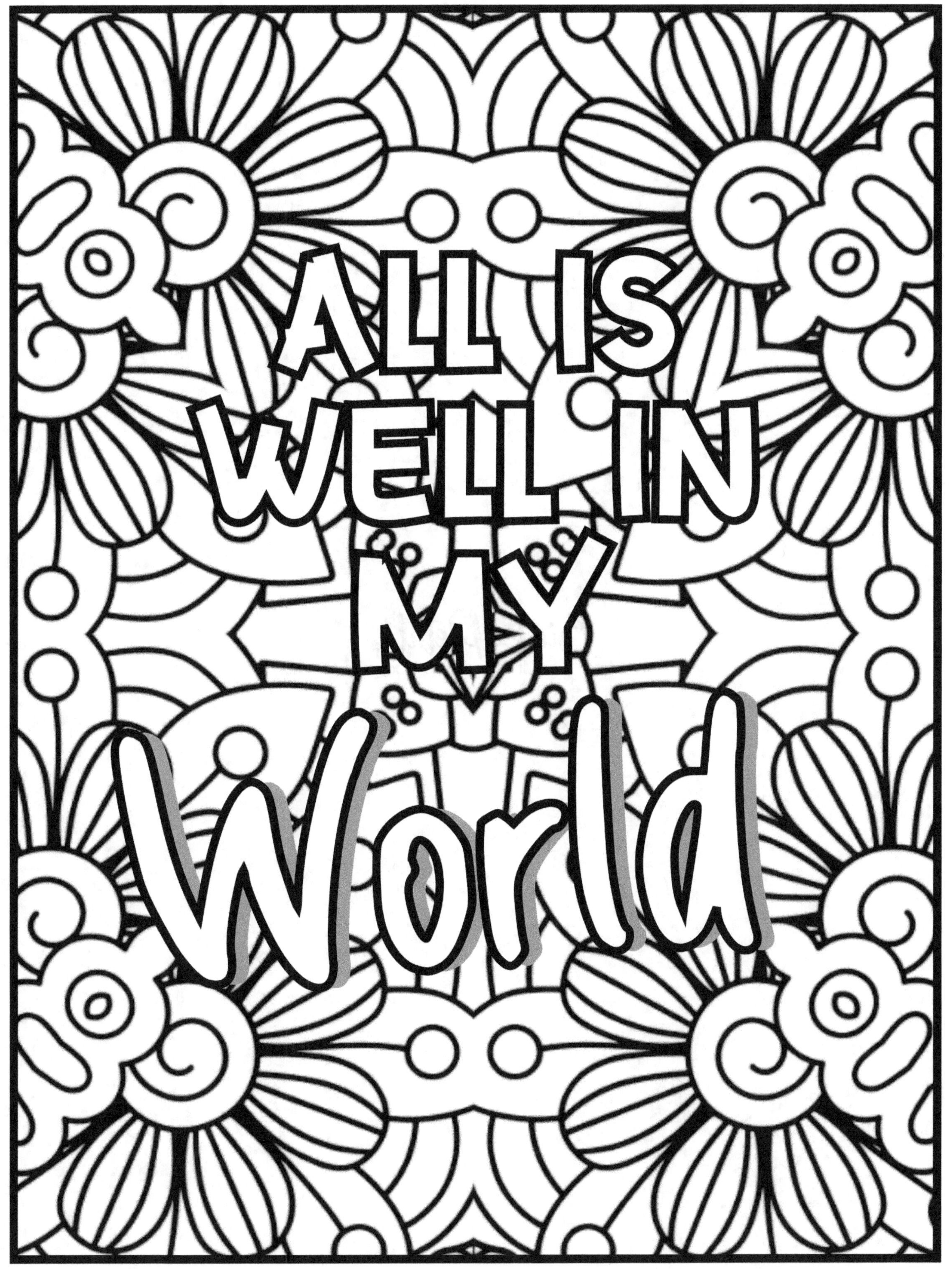

ALL IS
WELL IN
MY
World

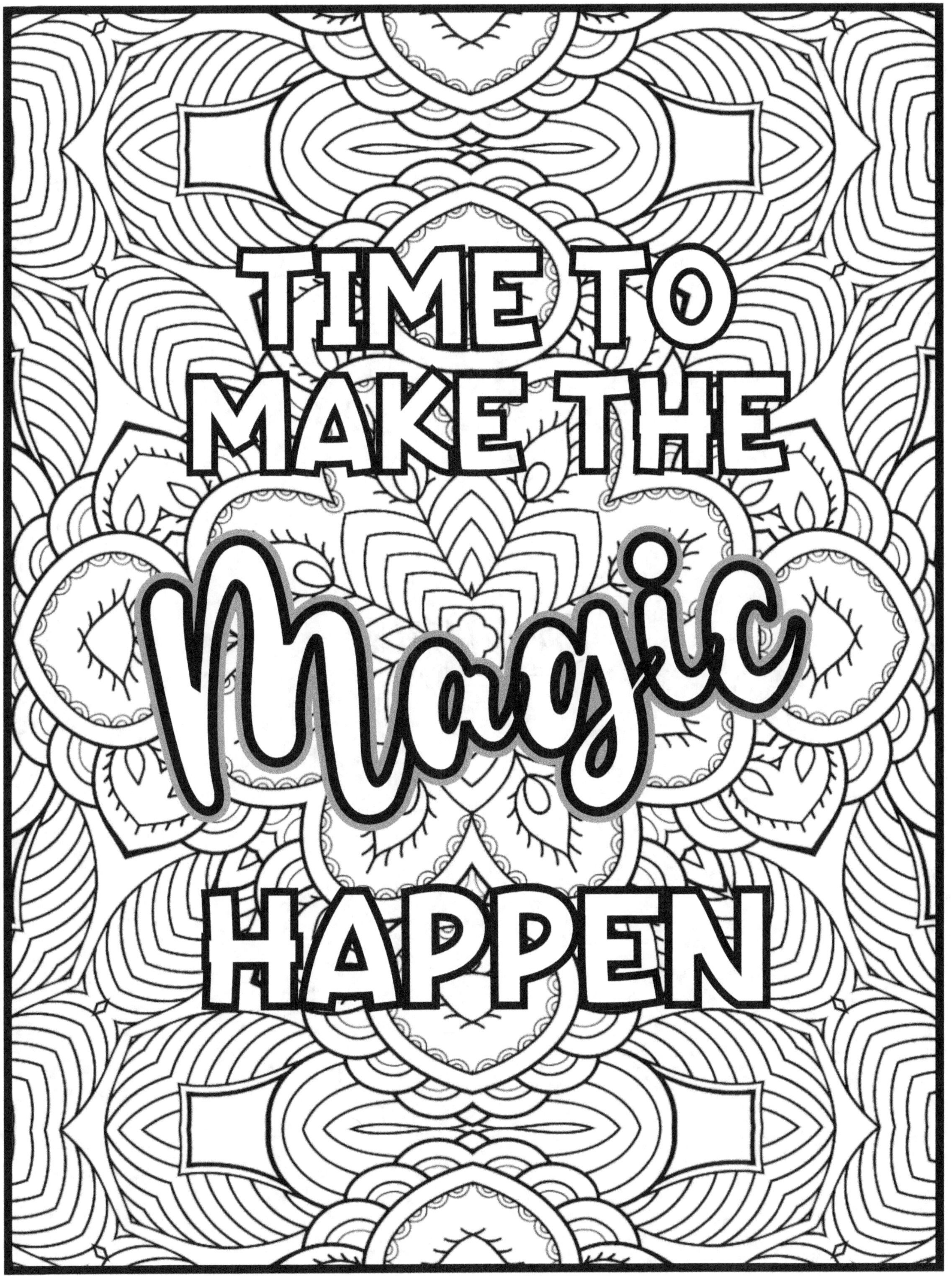

TIME TO
MAKE THE
Magic
HAPPEN

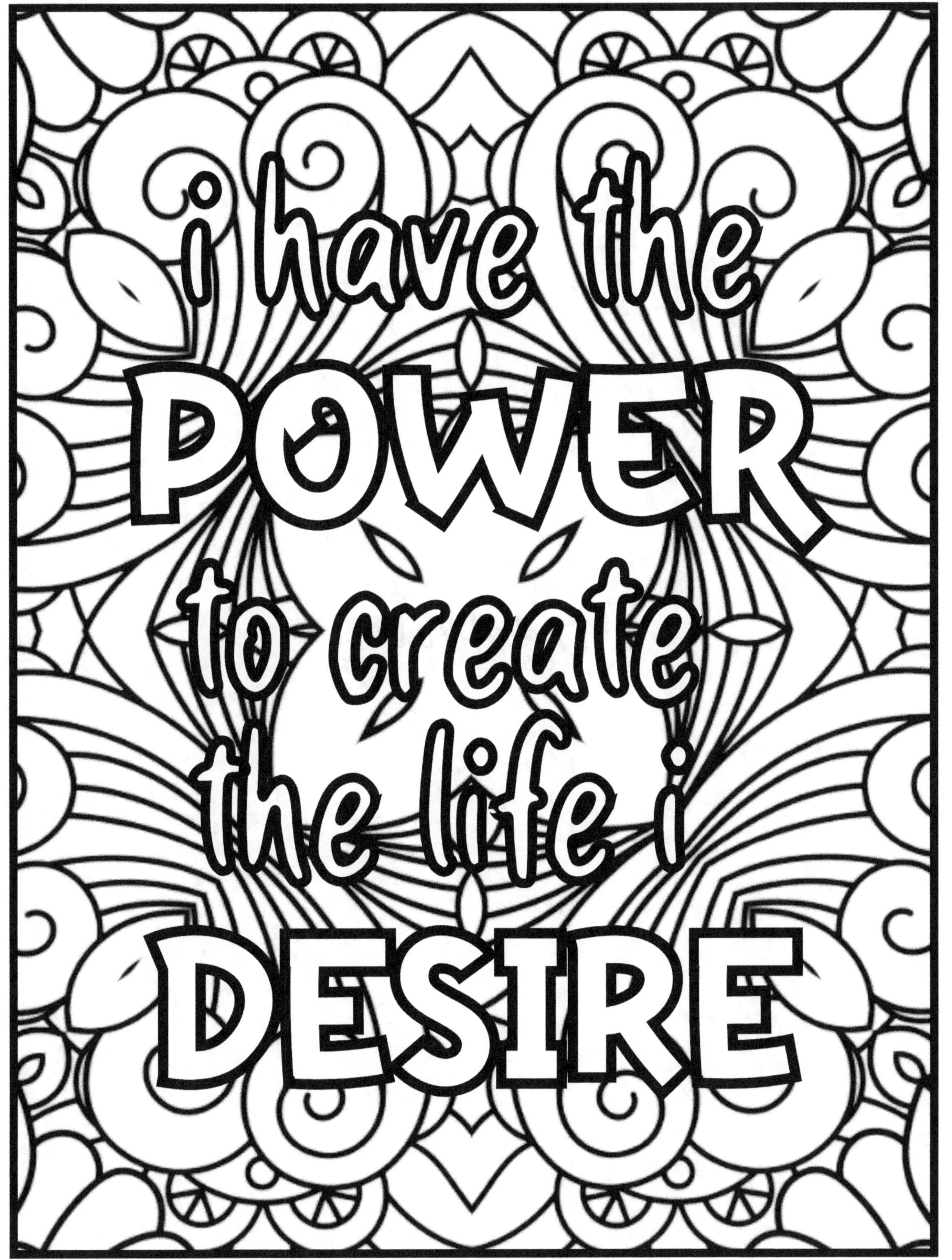

i have the
POWER
to create
the life i
DESIRE

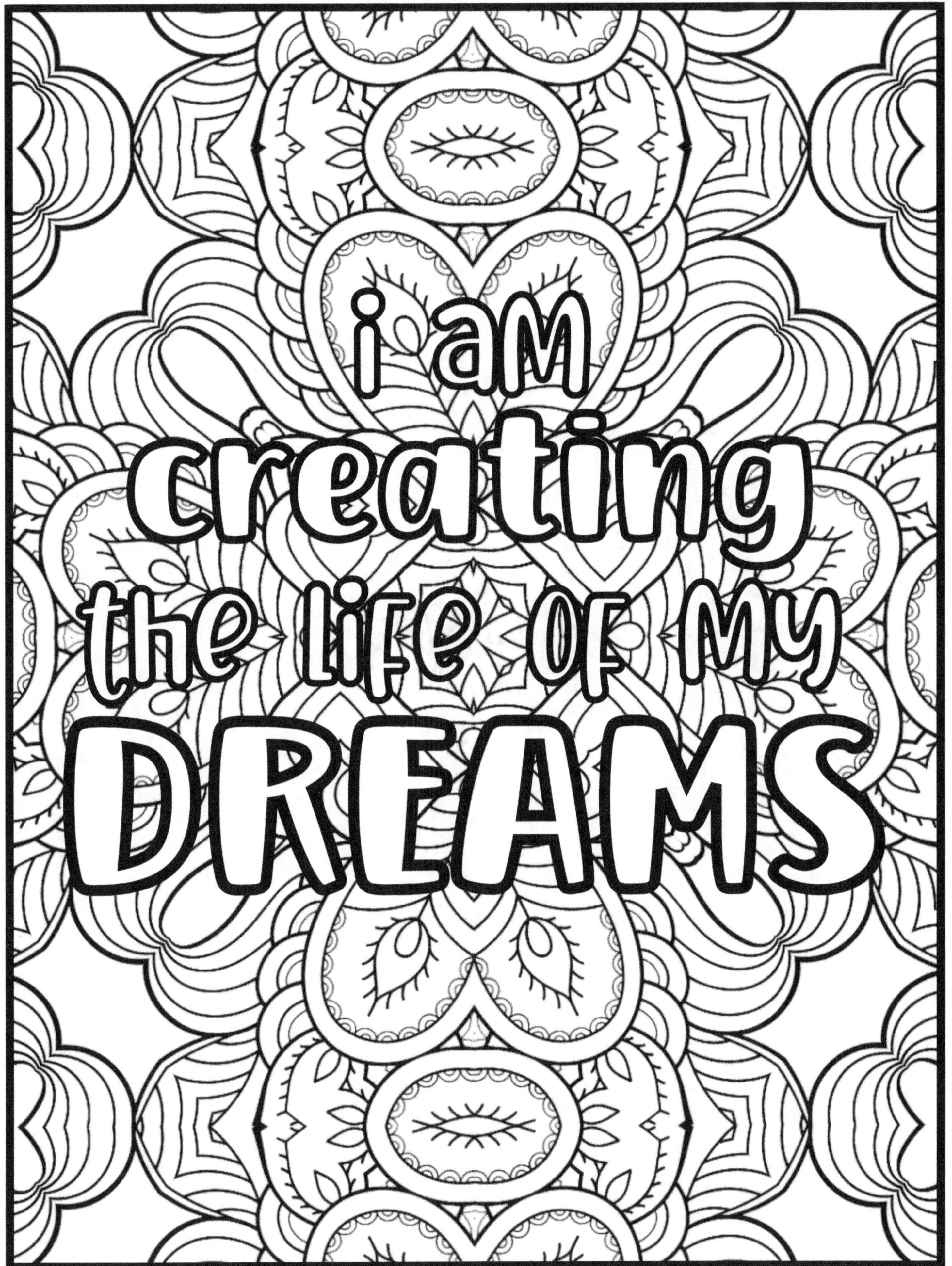

i am
creating
the life of my
DREAMS

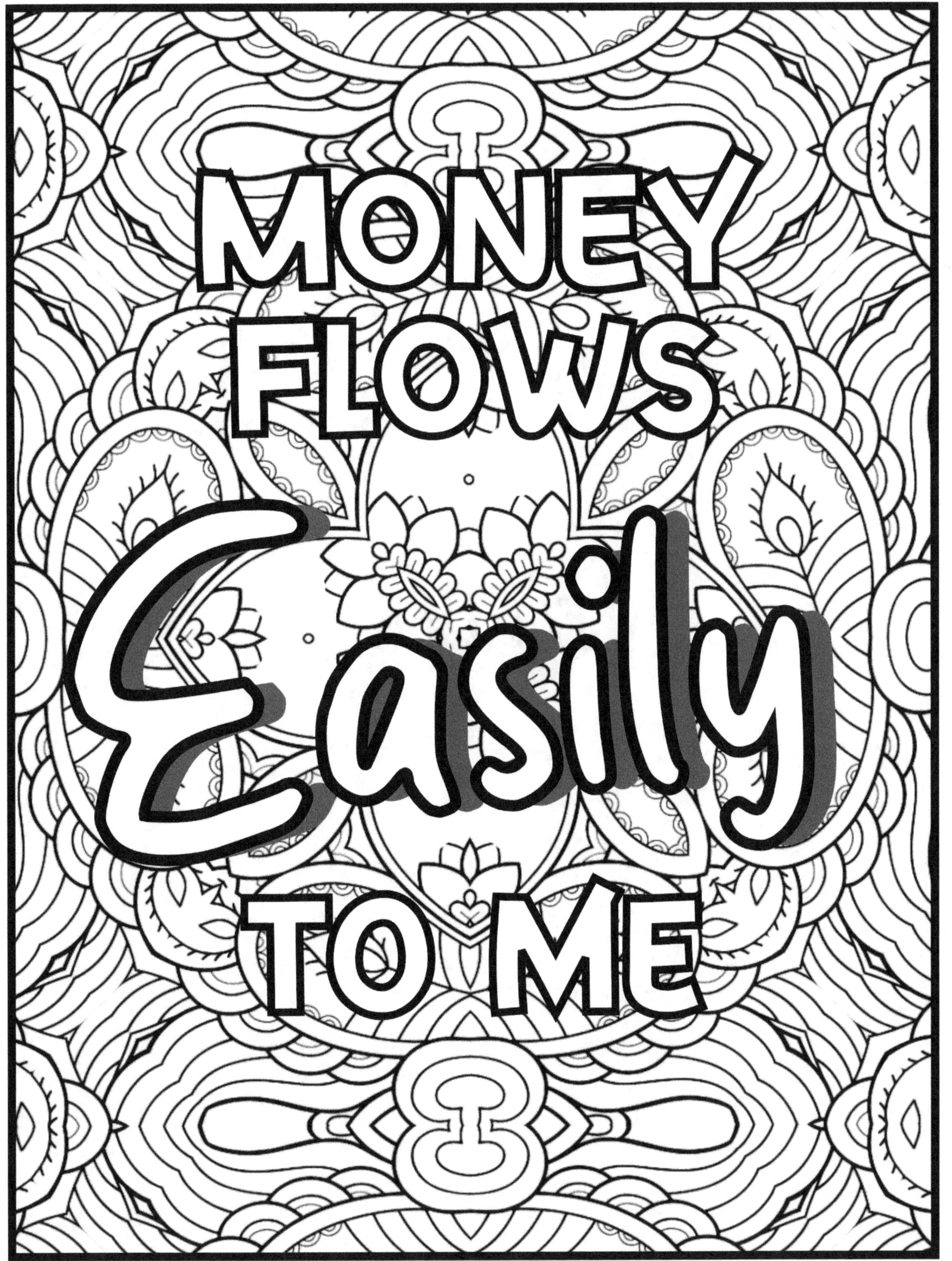

MONEY
FLOWS
Easily
TO ME

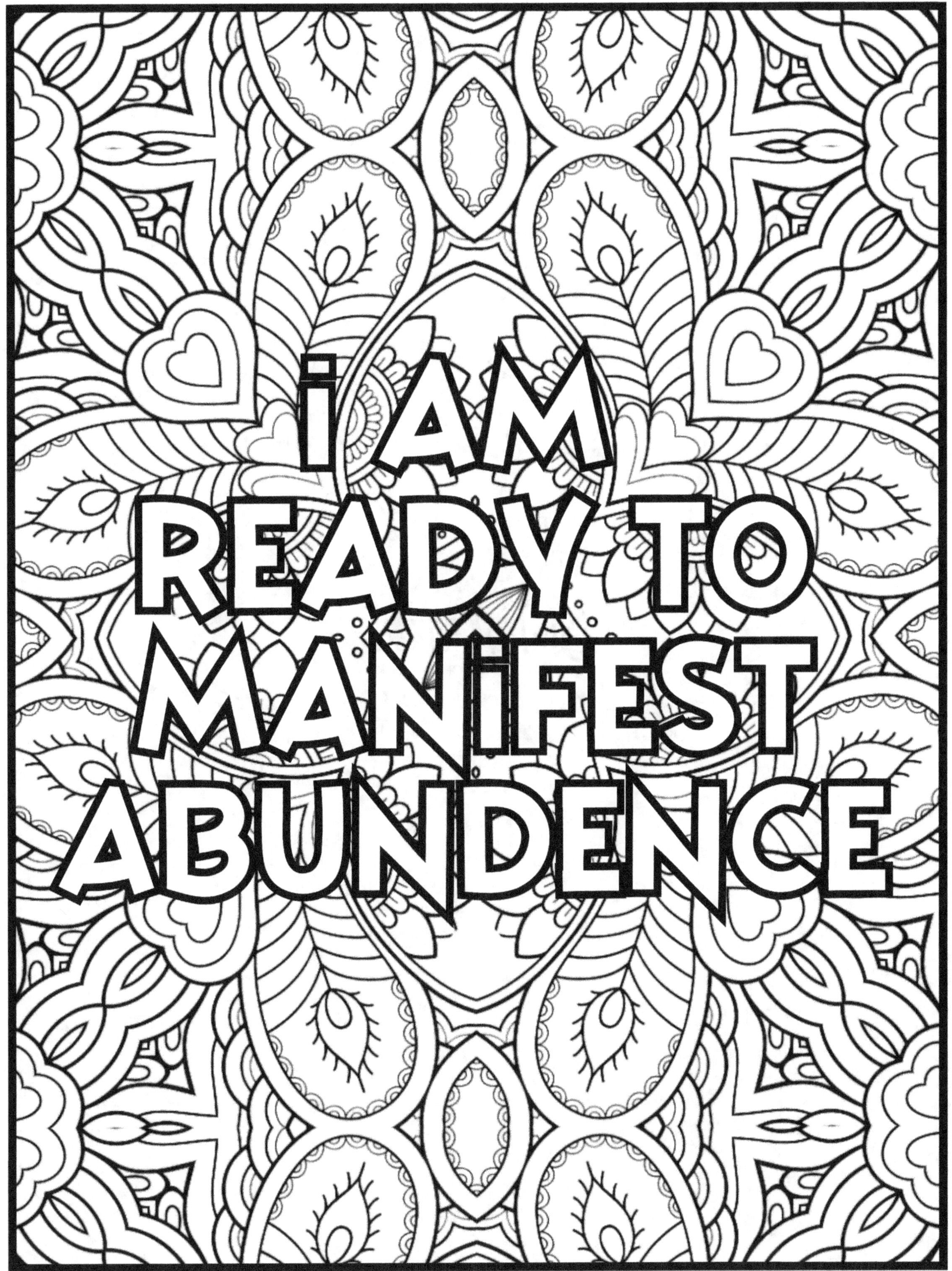

i AM
READY TO
MANIFEST
ABUNDENCE

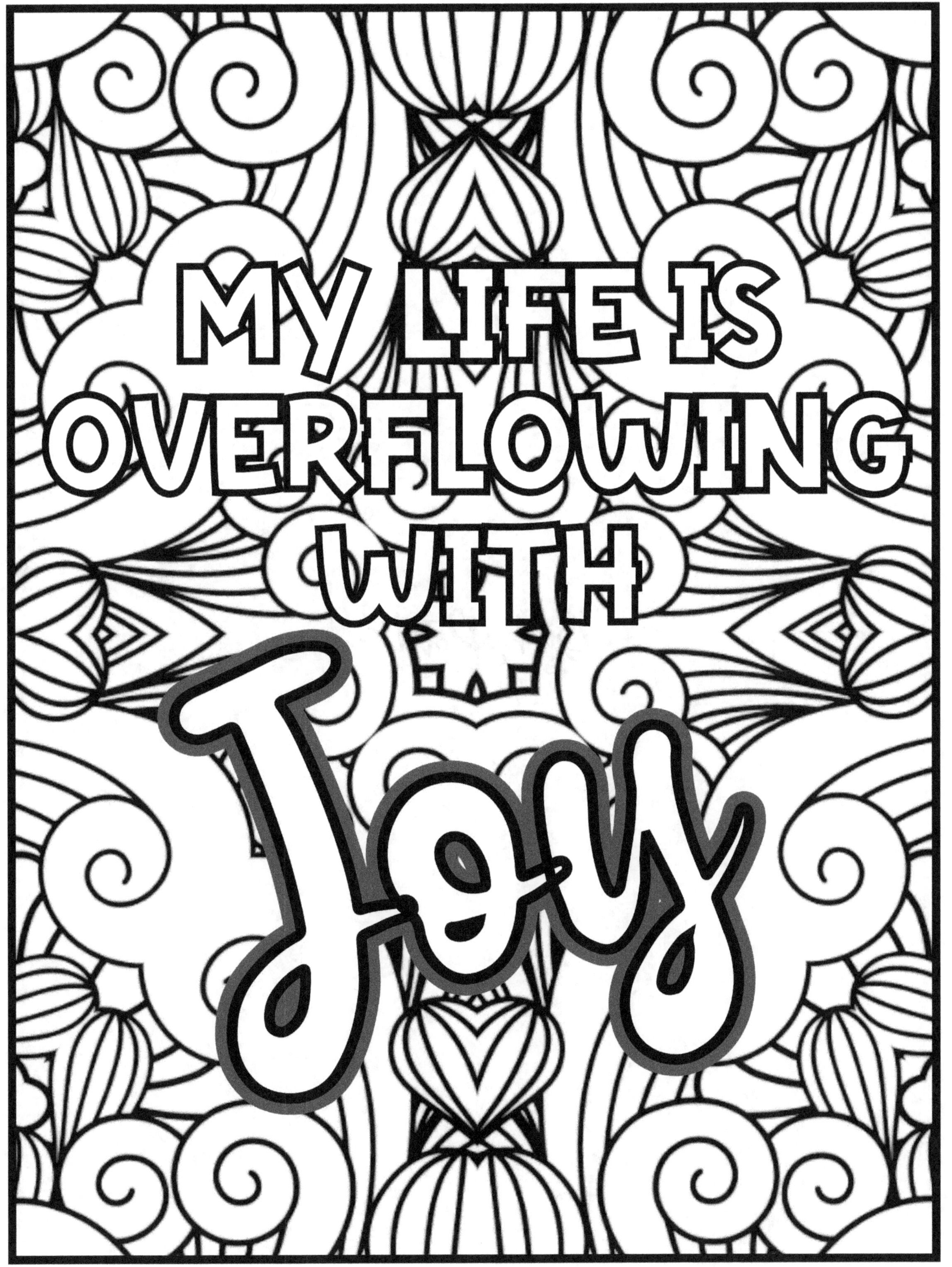

MY LIFE IS
OVERFLOWING
WITH
Joy

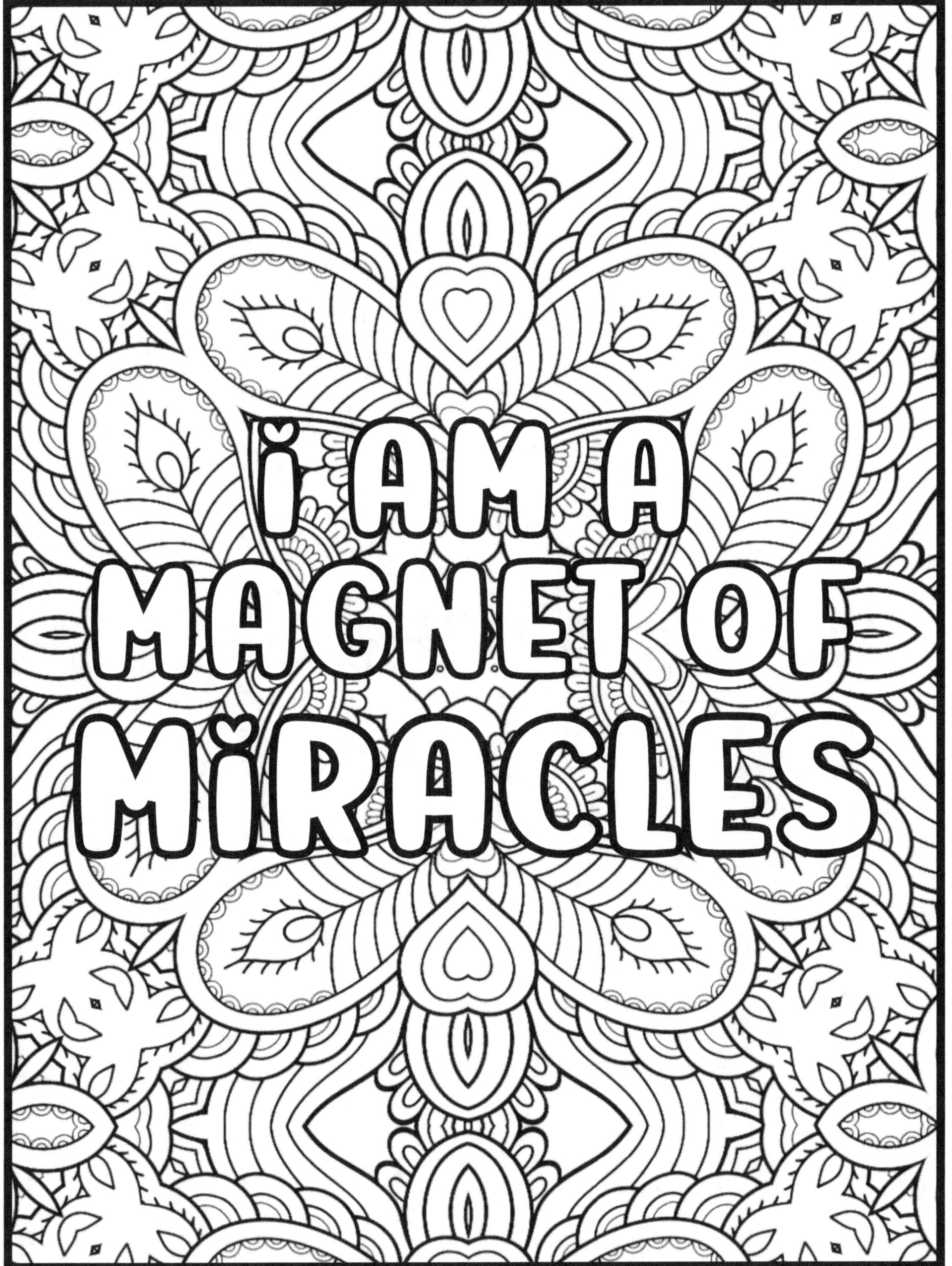

I AM A MAGNET OF MIRACLES

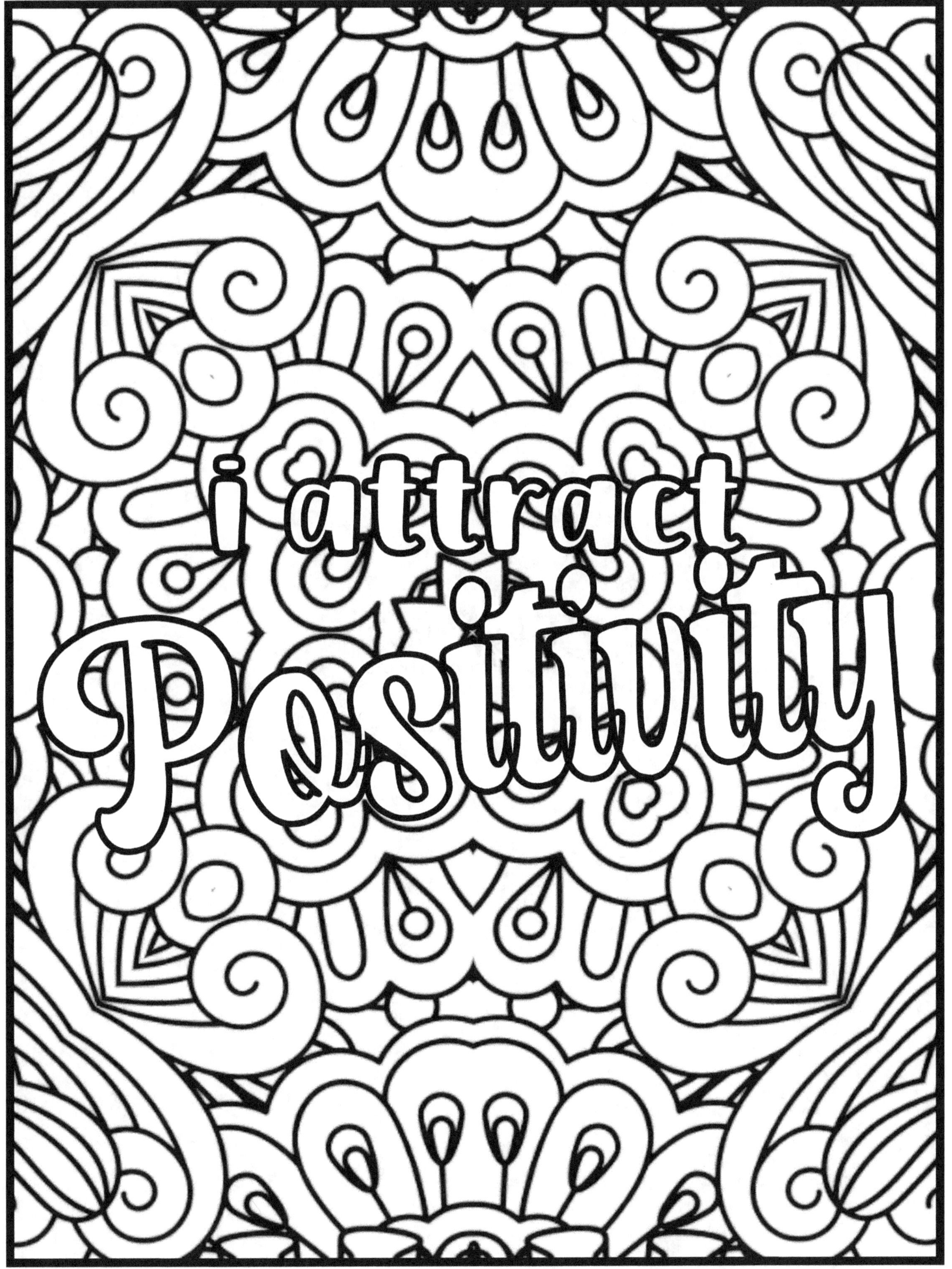

i attract
Positivity

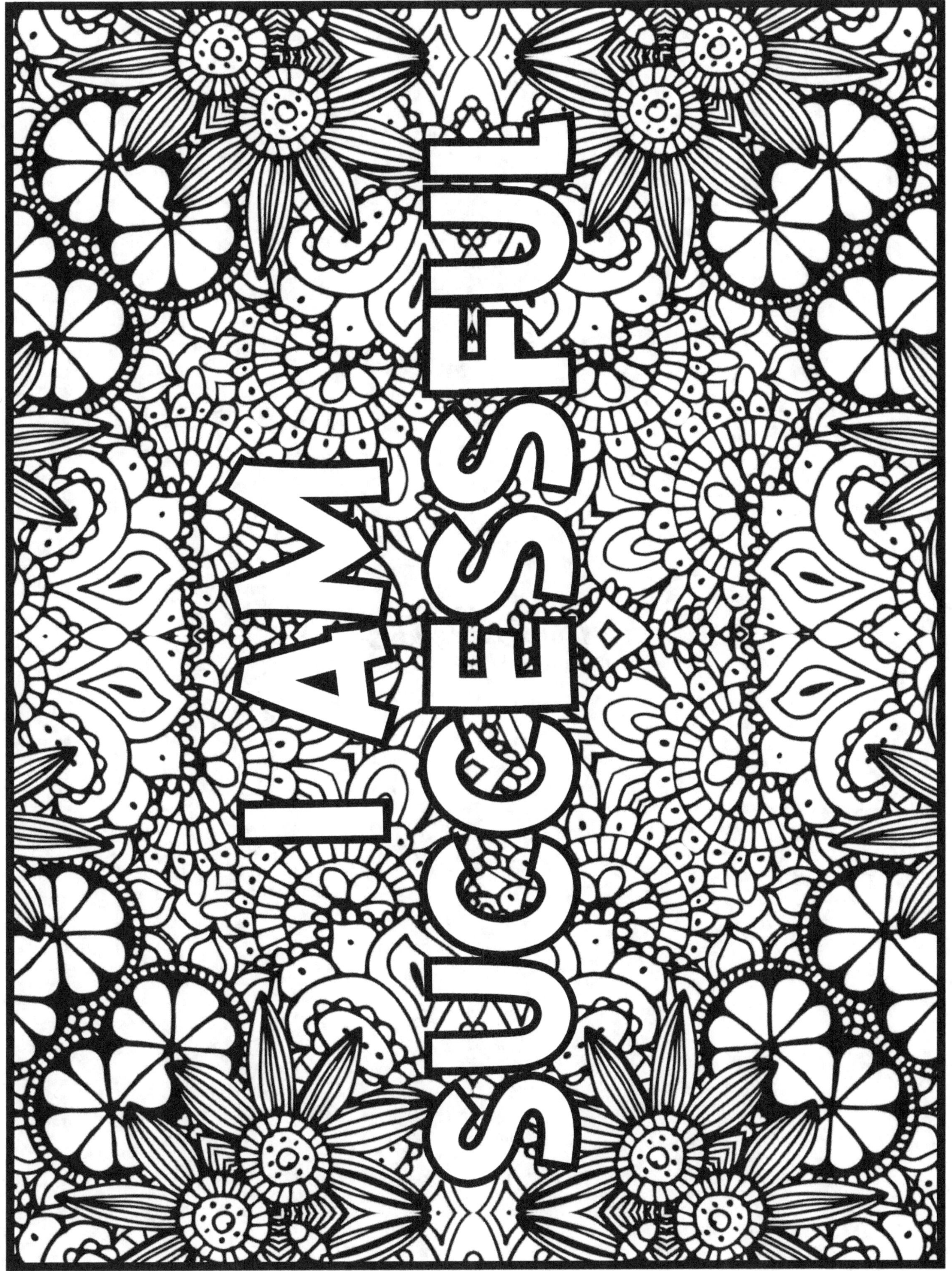

I AM SUCCESSFUL

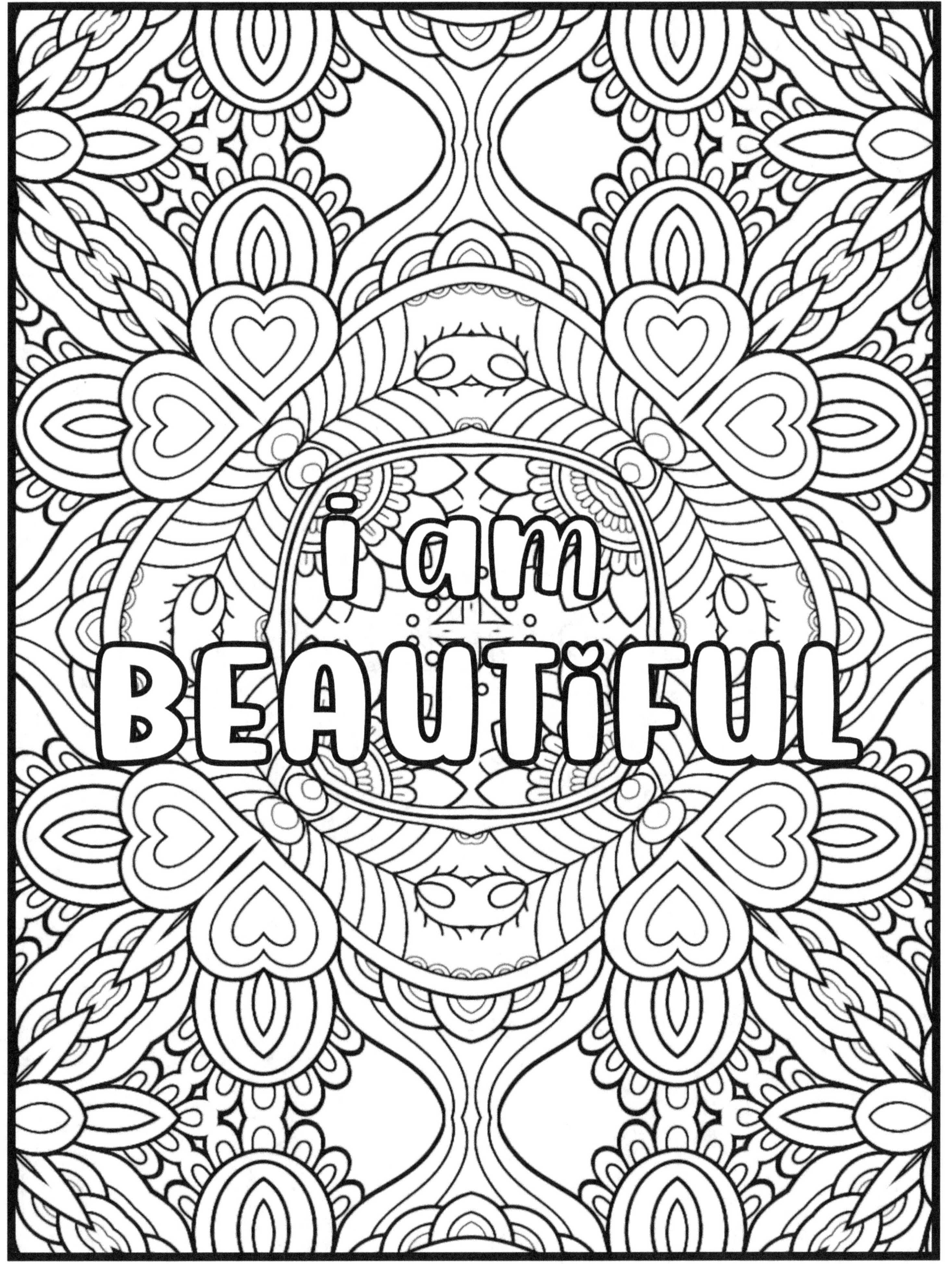

i am
BEAUTiFUL

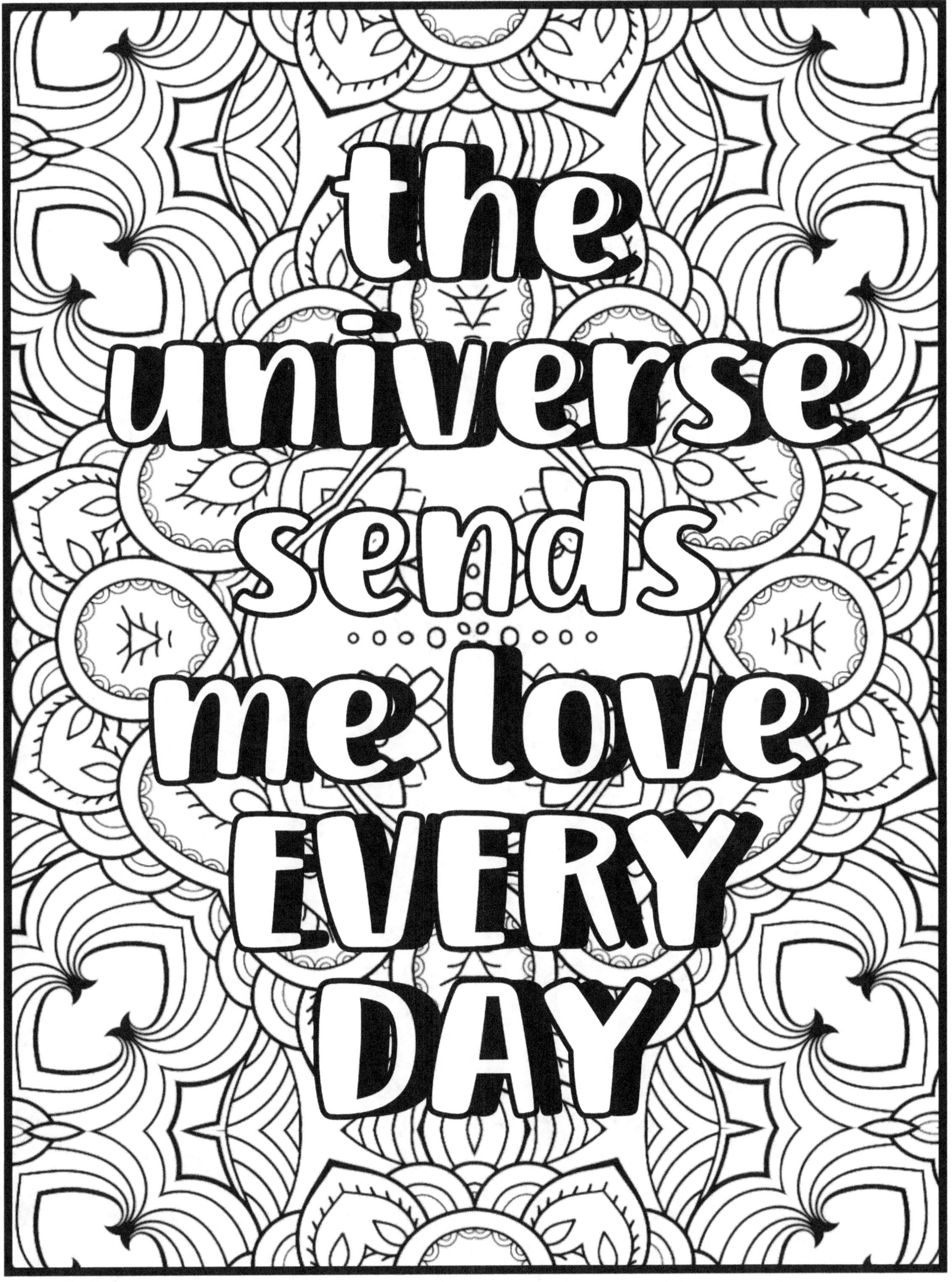

the
universe
sends
me love
EVERY
DAY

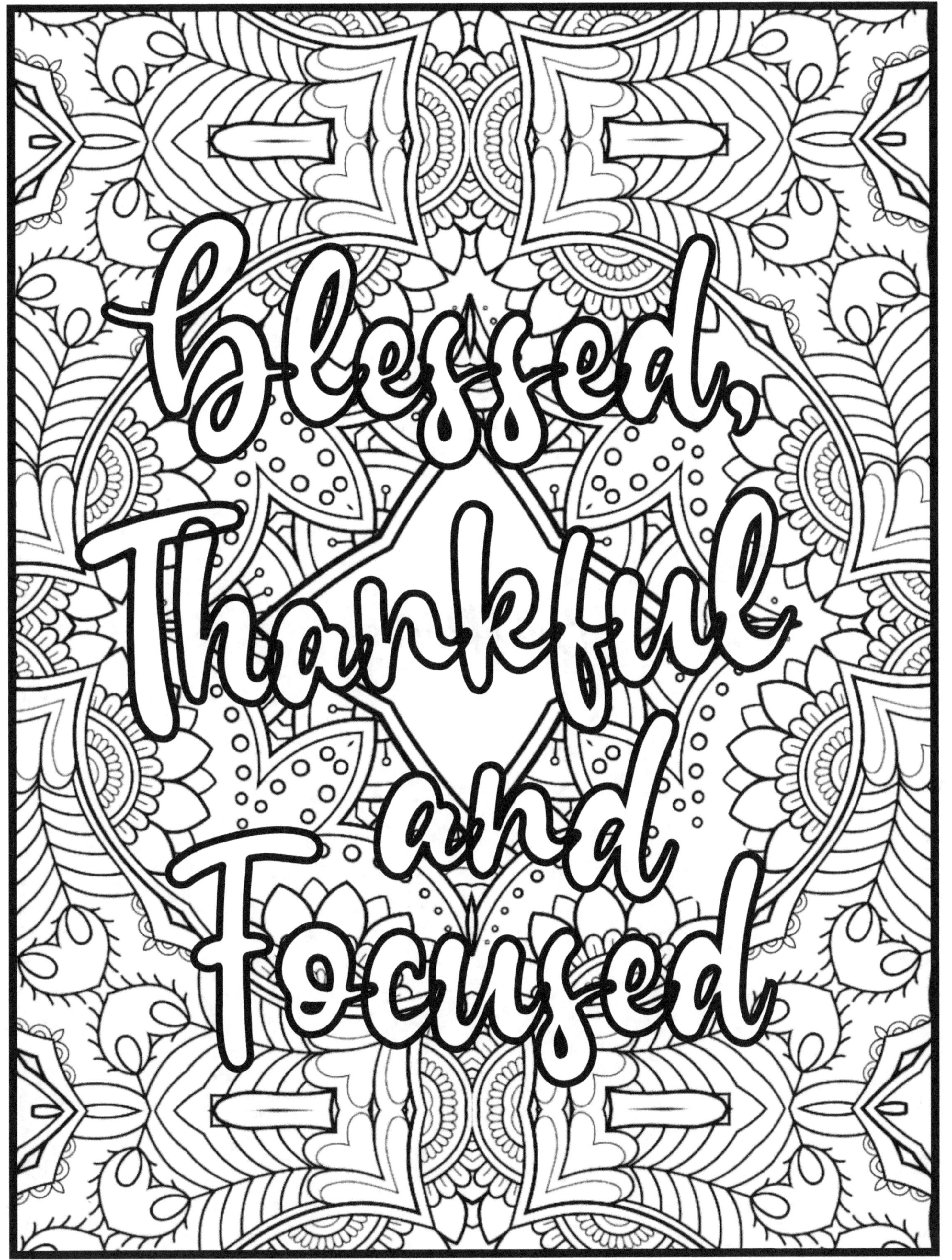
blessed,
Thankful
and
Focused

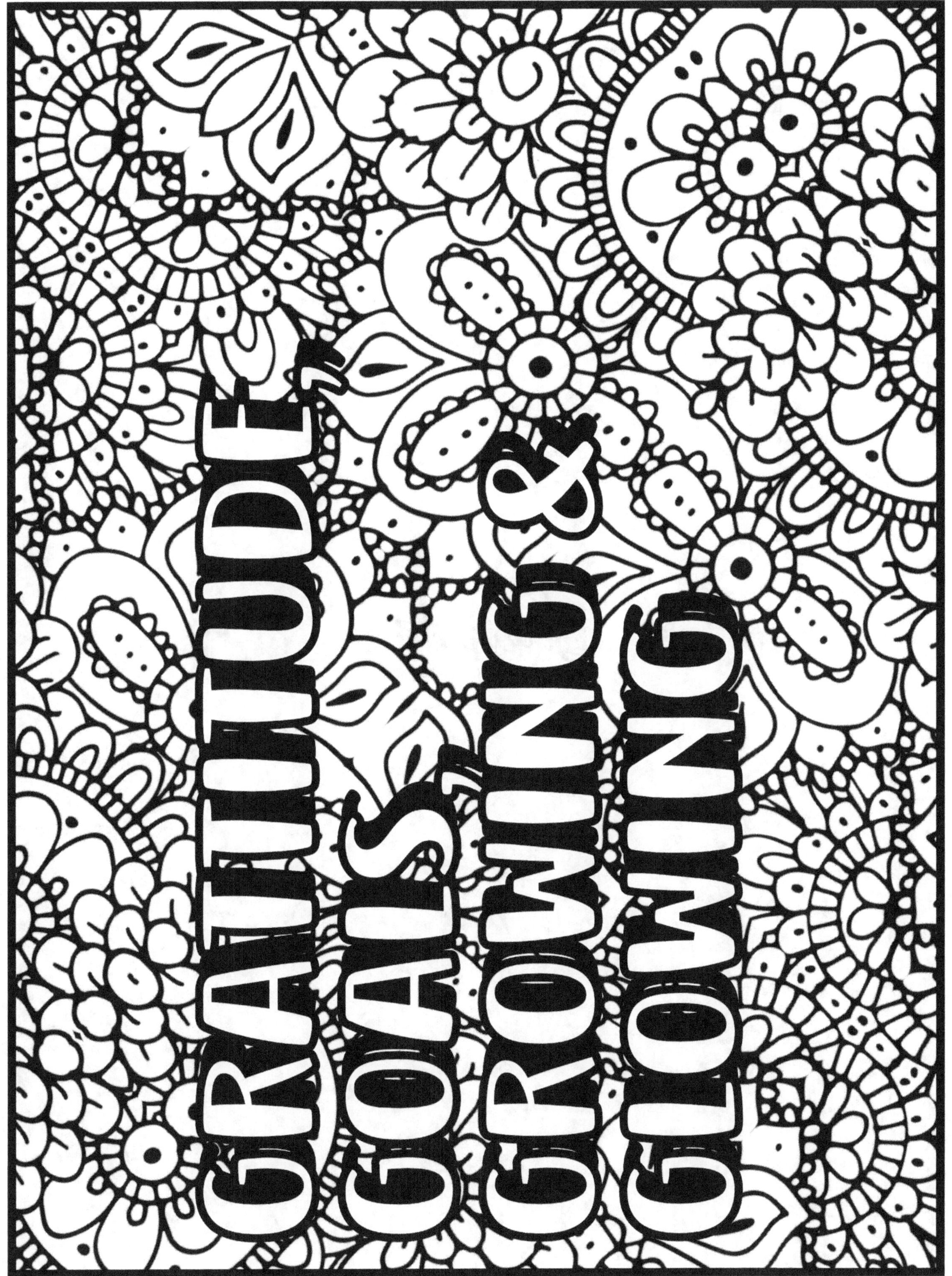

GRATITUDE,
GOALS,
GROWING &
GLOWING

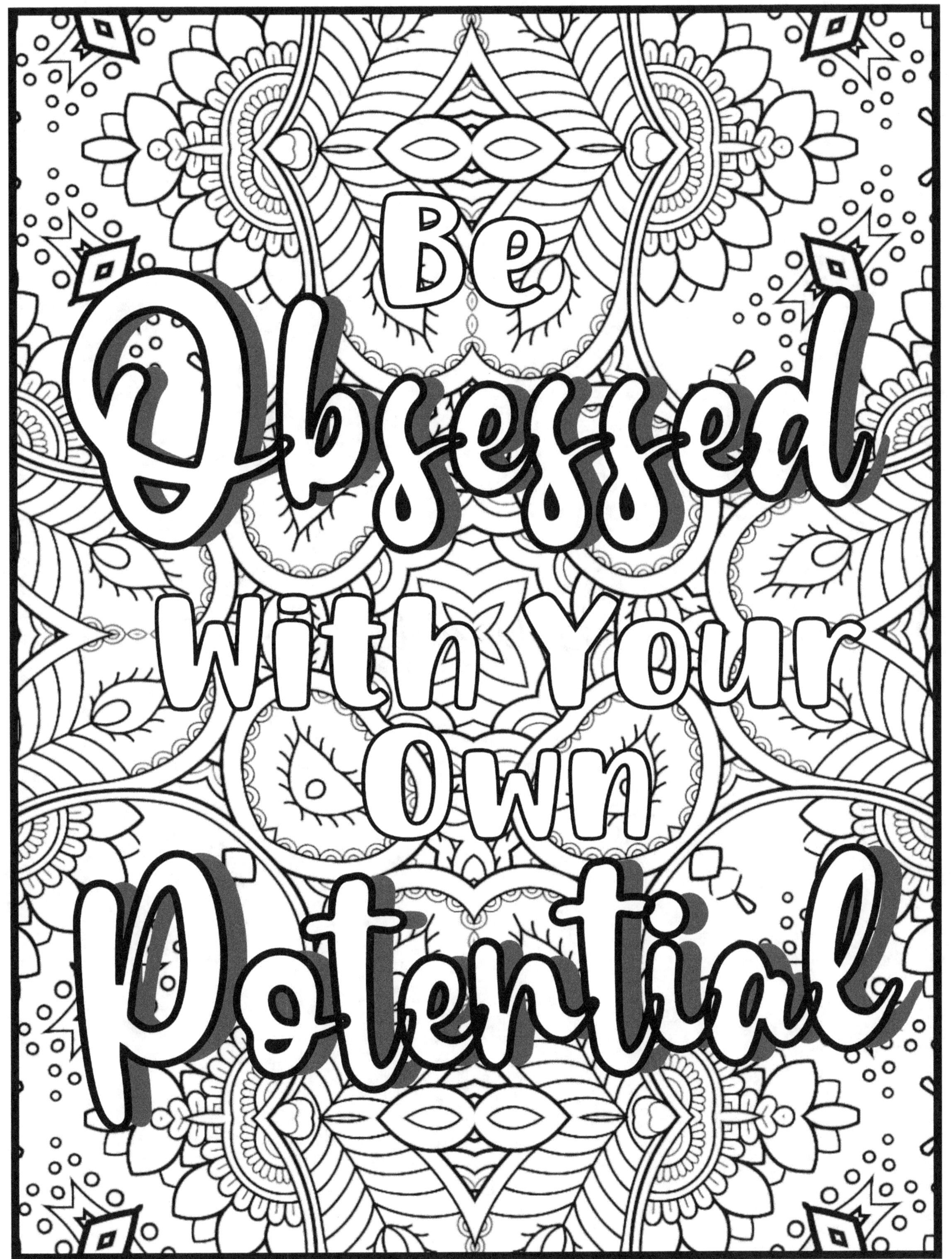

Be
Obsessed
With Your
Own
Potential

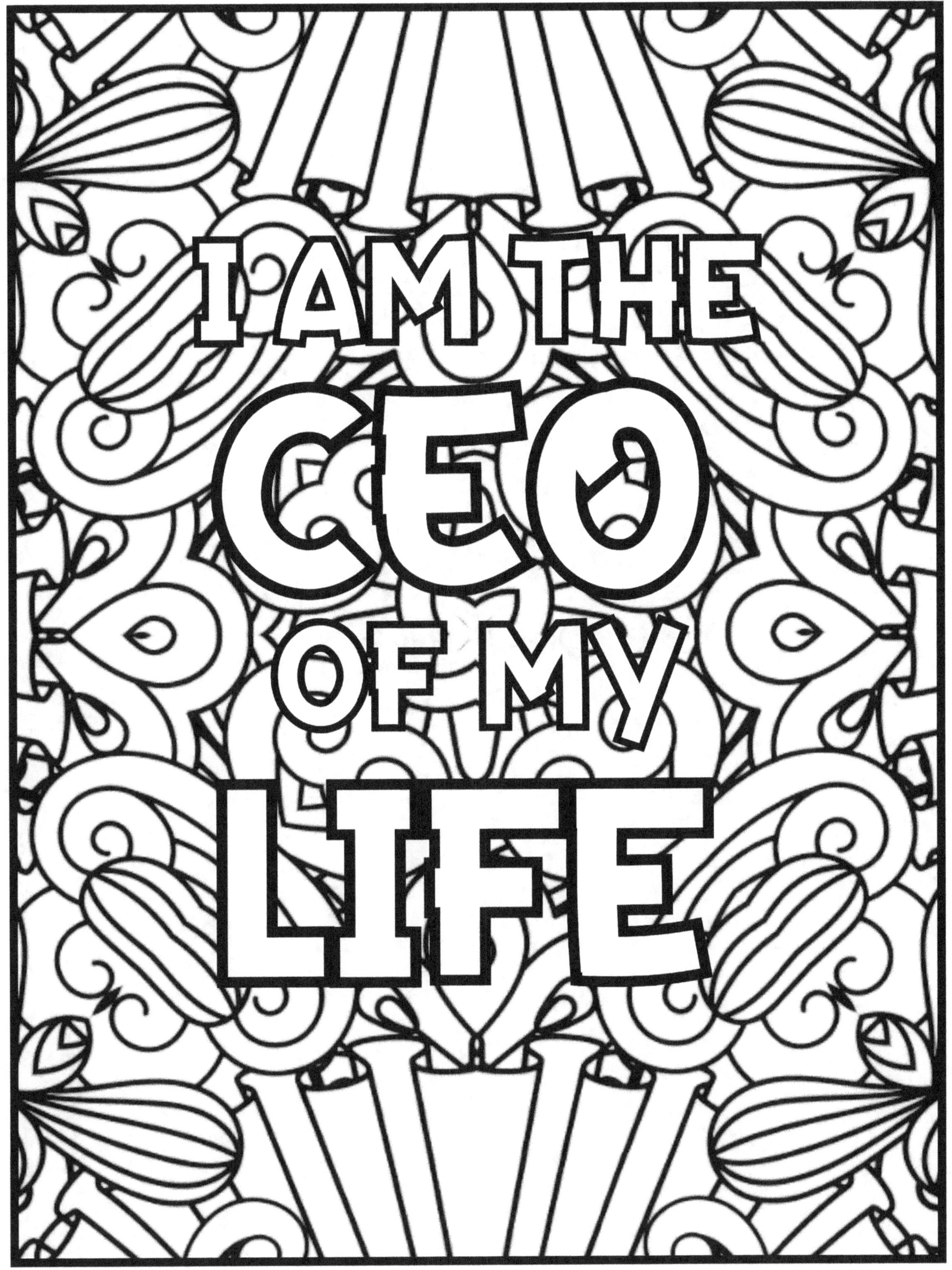
I AM THE
CEO
OF MY
LIFE

BinkyPetal's
adult coloring books

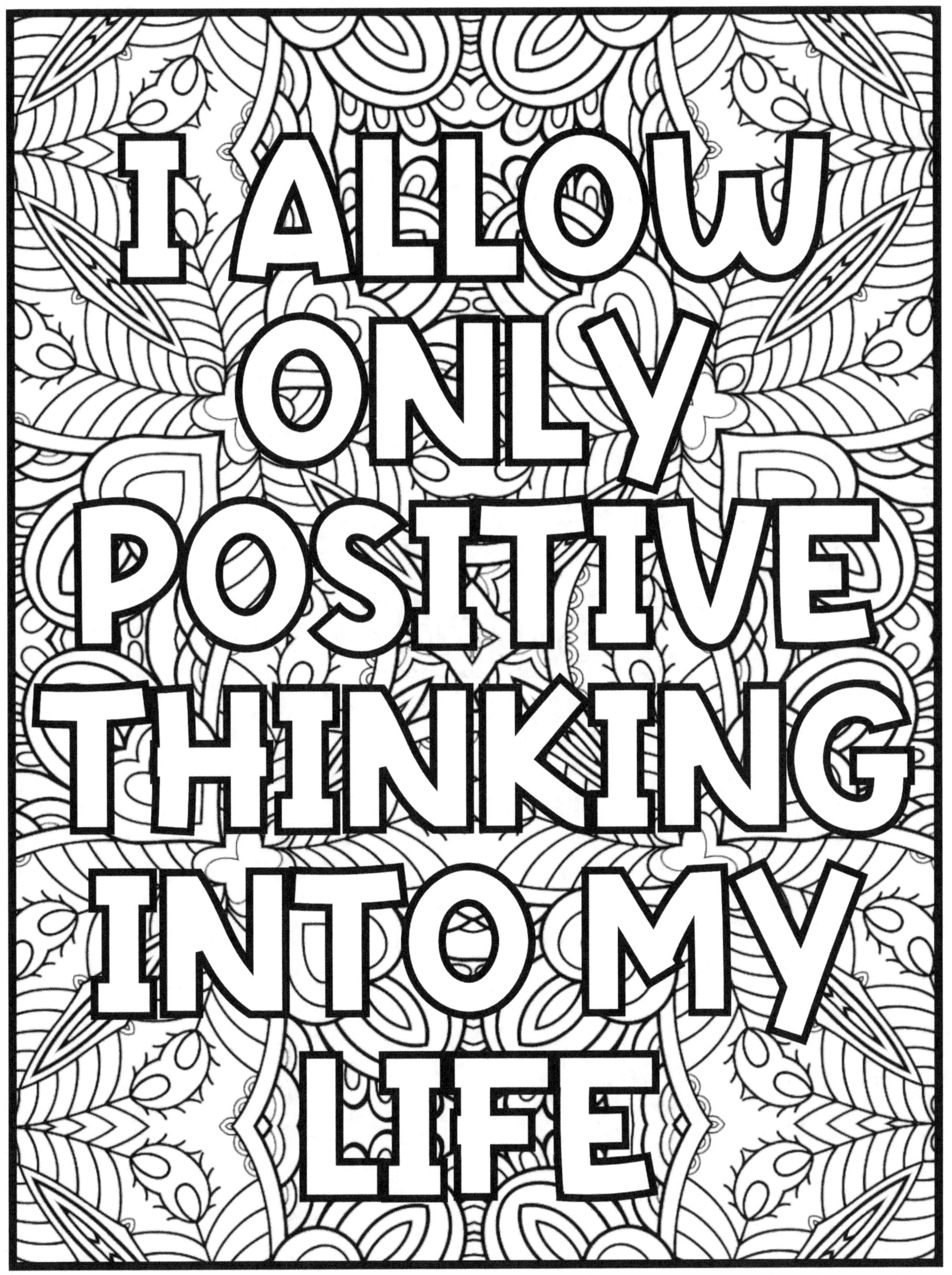

I ALLOW ONLY POSITIVE THINKING INTO MY LIFE

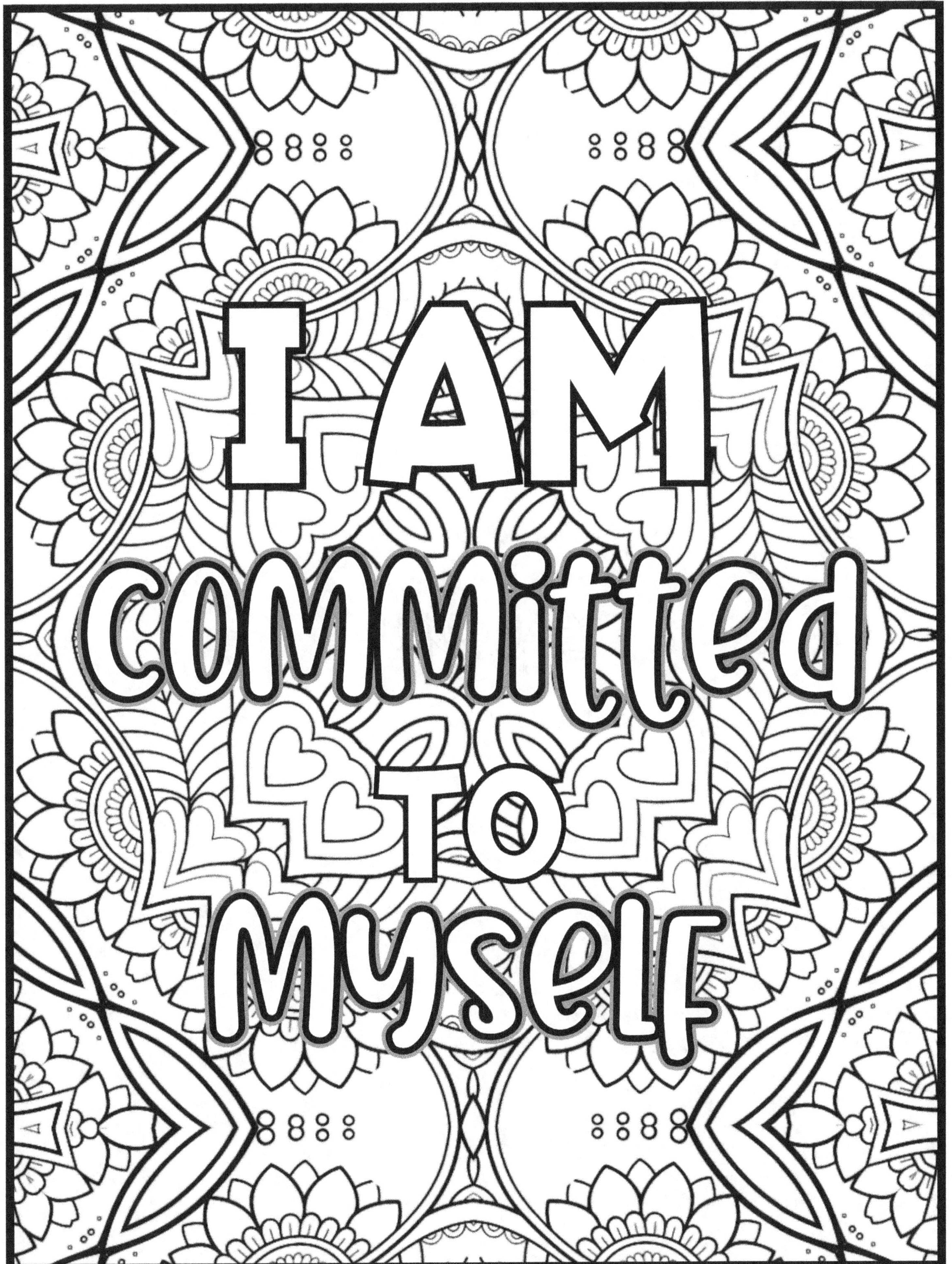

I AM
committed
to
Myself

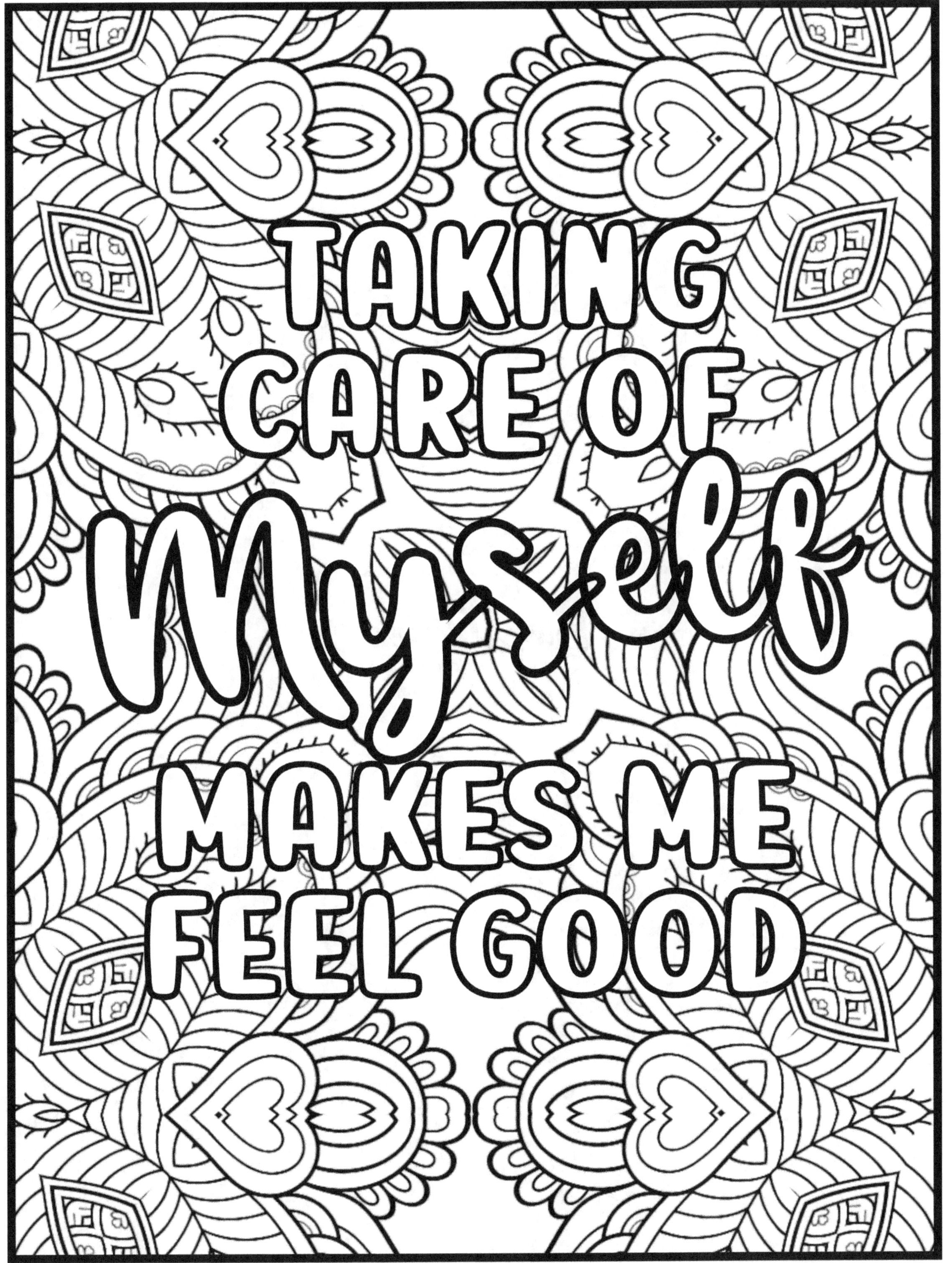

TAKING
CARE OF
Myself
MAKES ME
FEEL GOOD

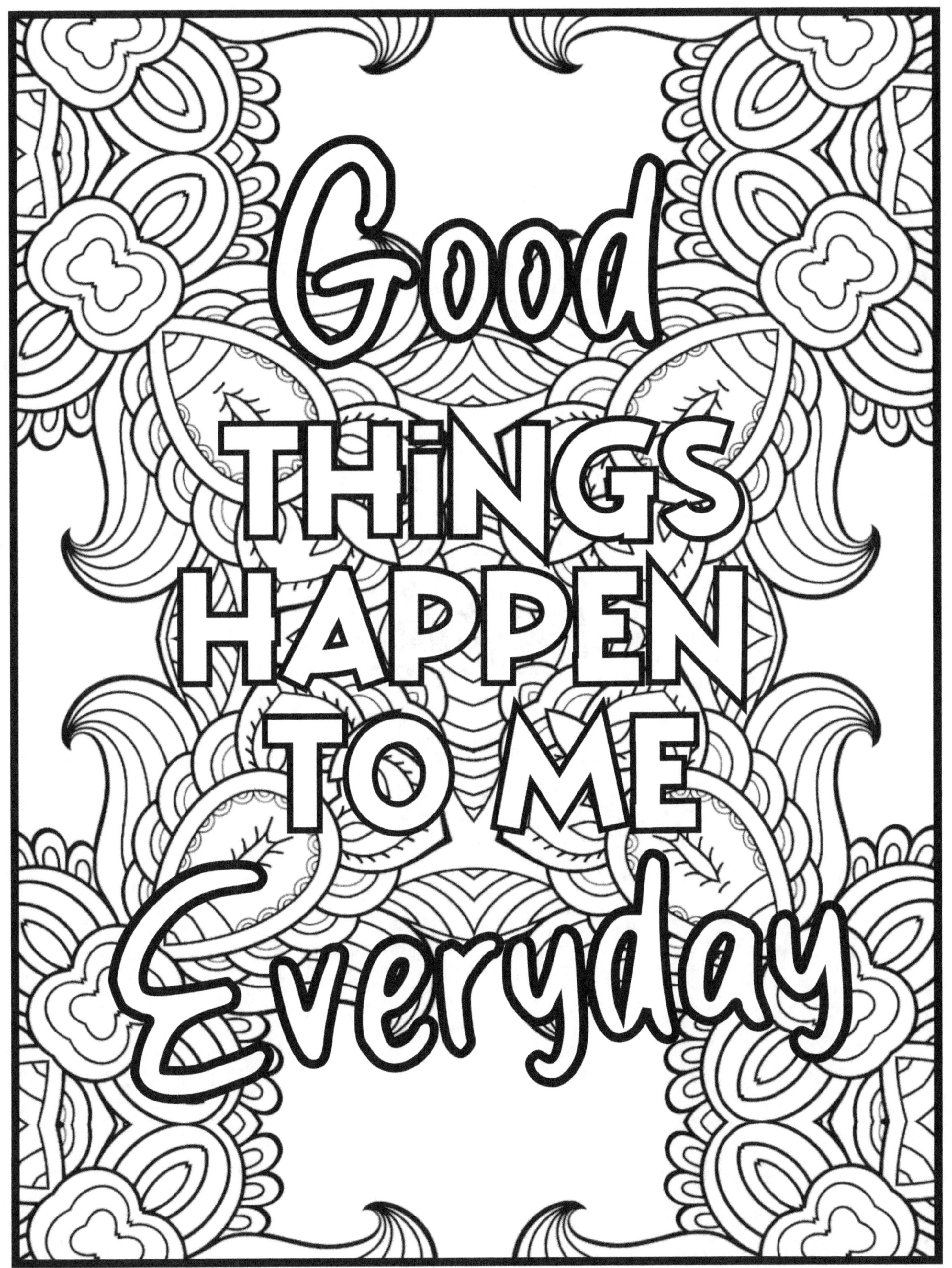
Good
THiNGS
HAPPEN
TO ME
Everyday

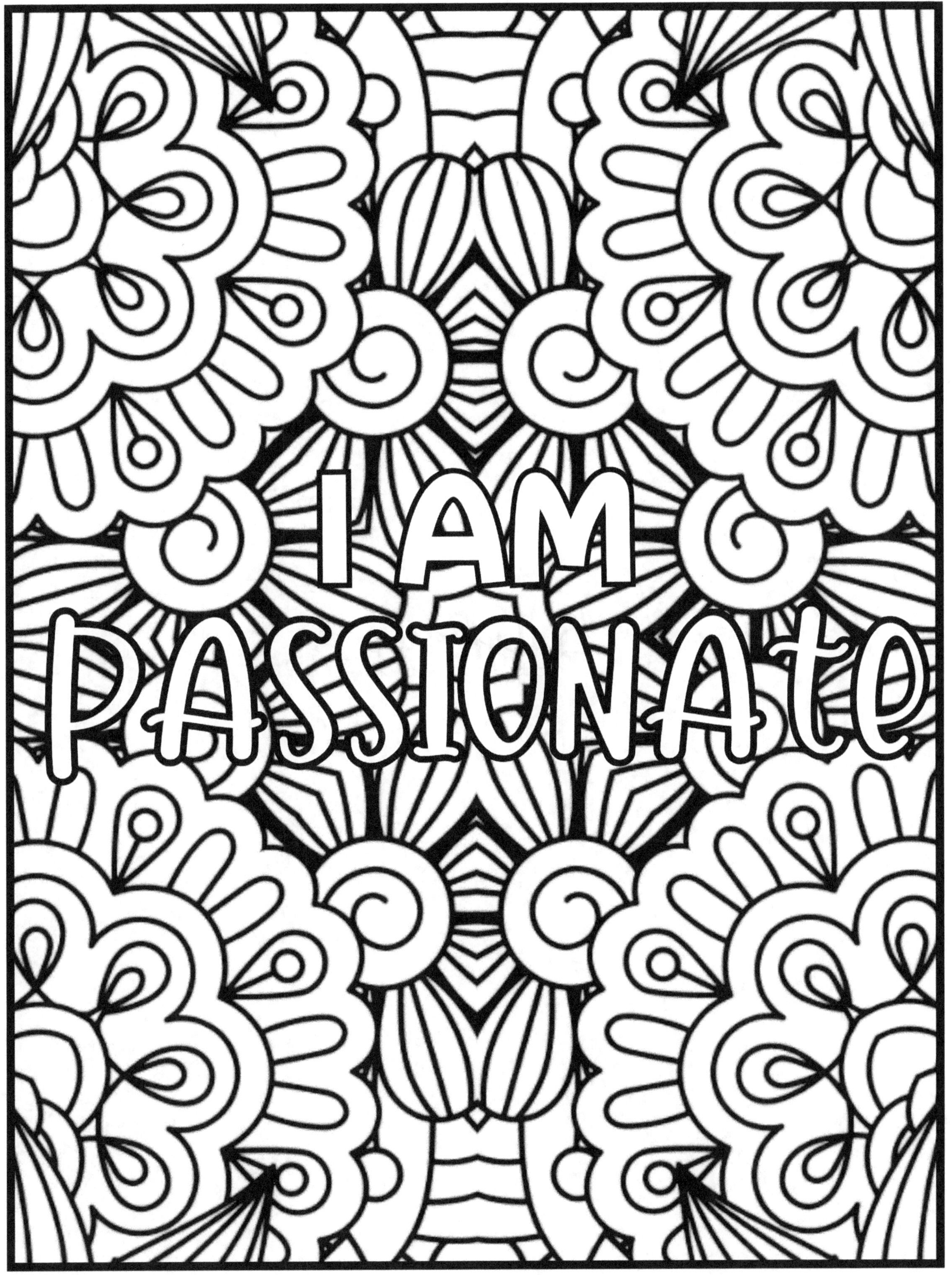

I AM
PASSIONATE

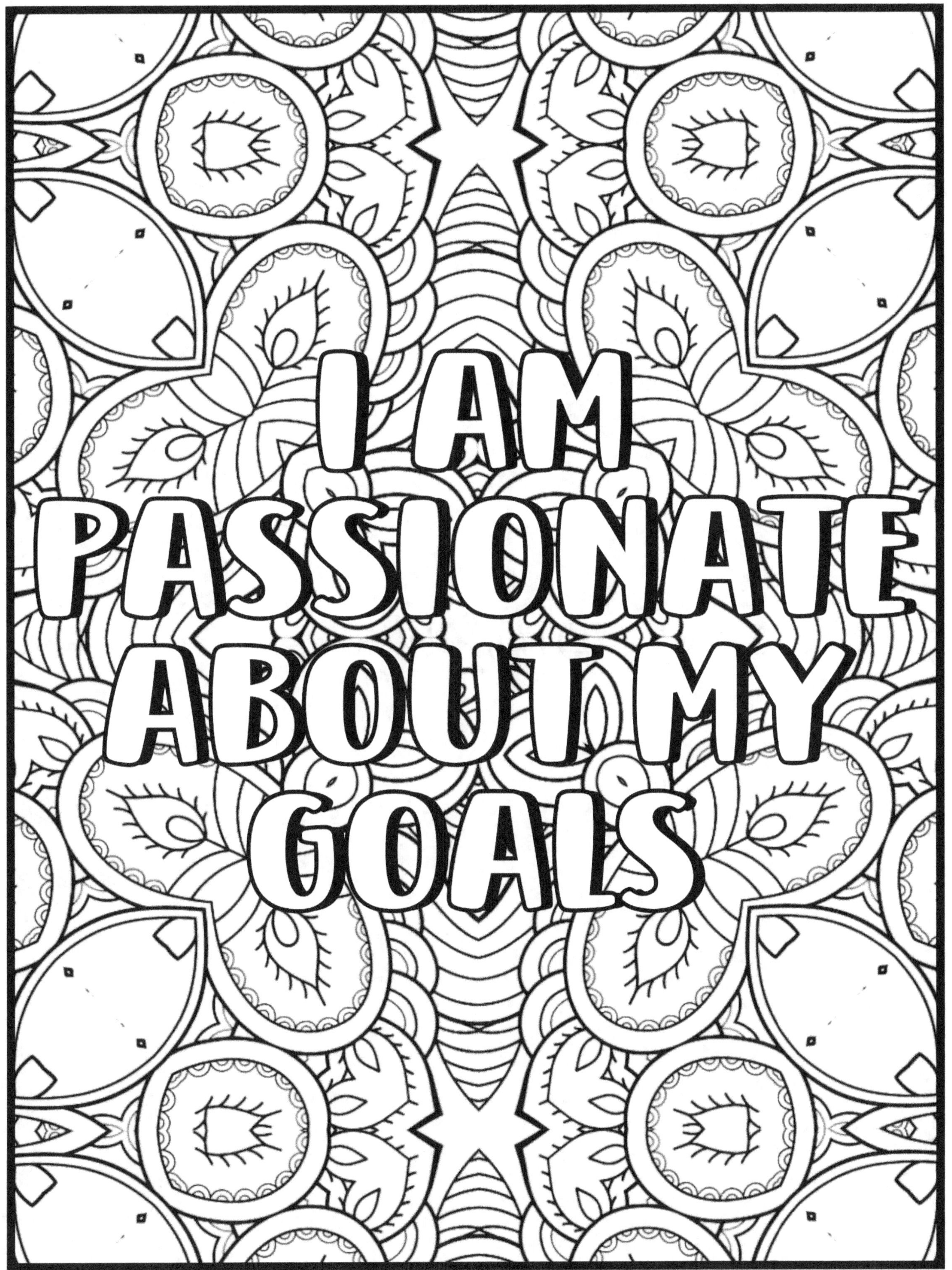

I AM
PASSIONATE
ABOUT MY
GOALS

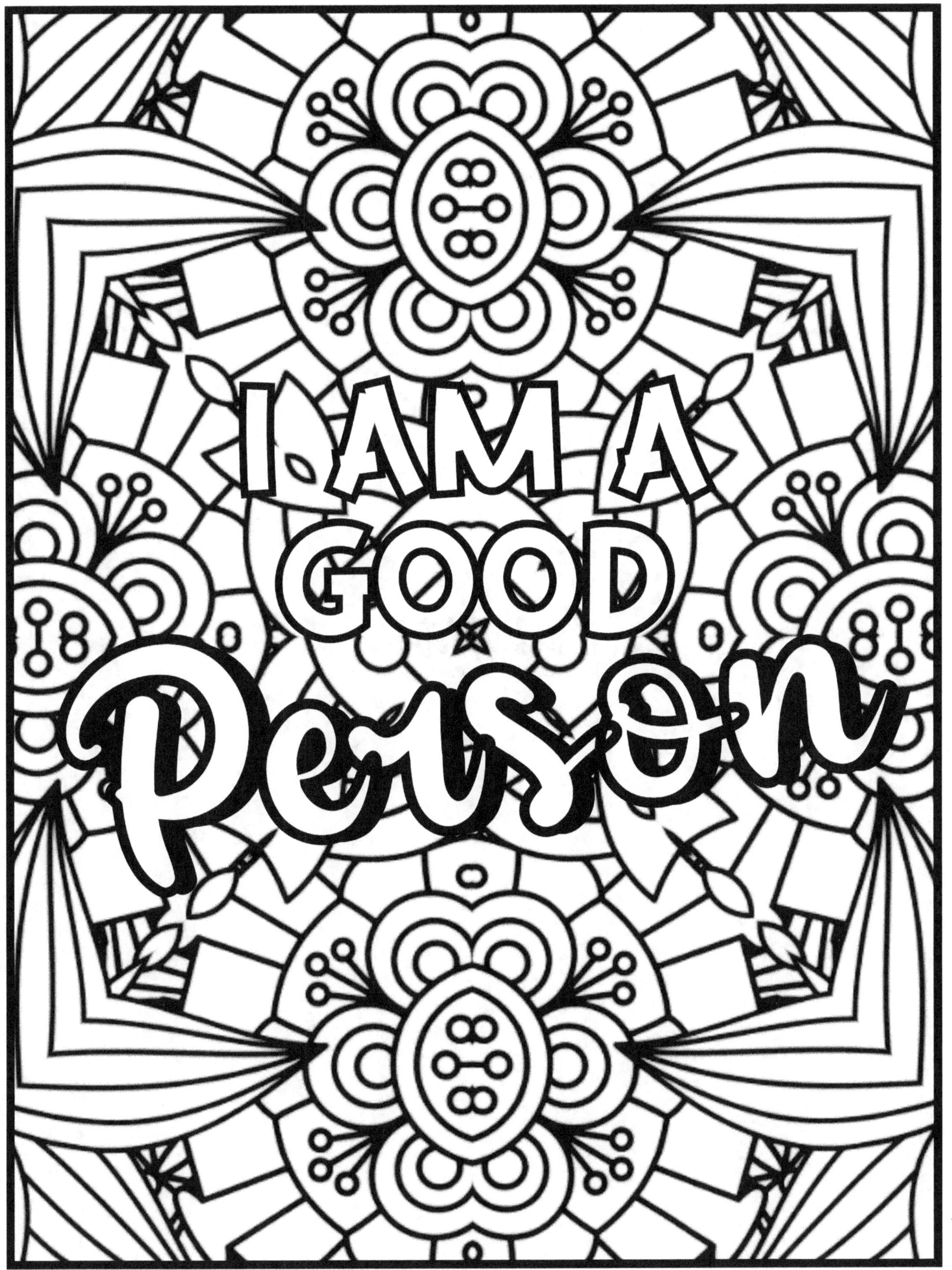

I AM A
GOOD
Person

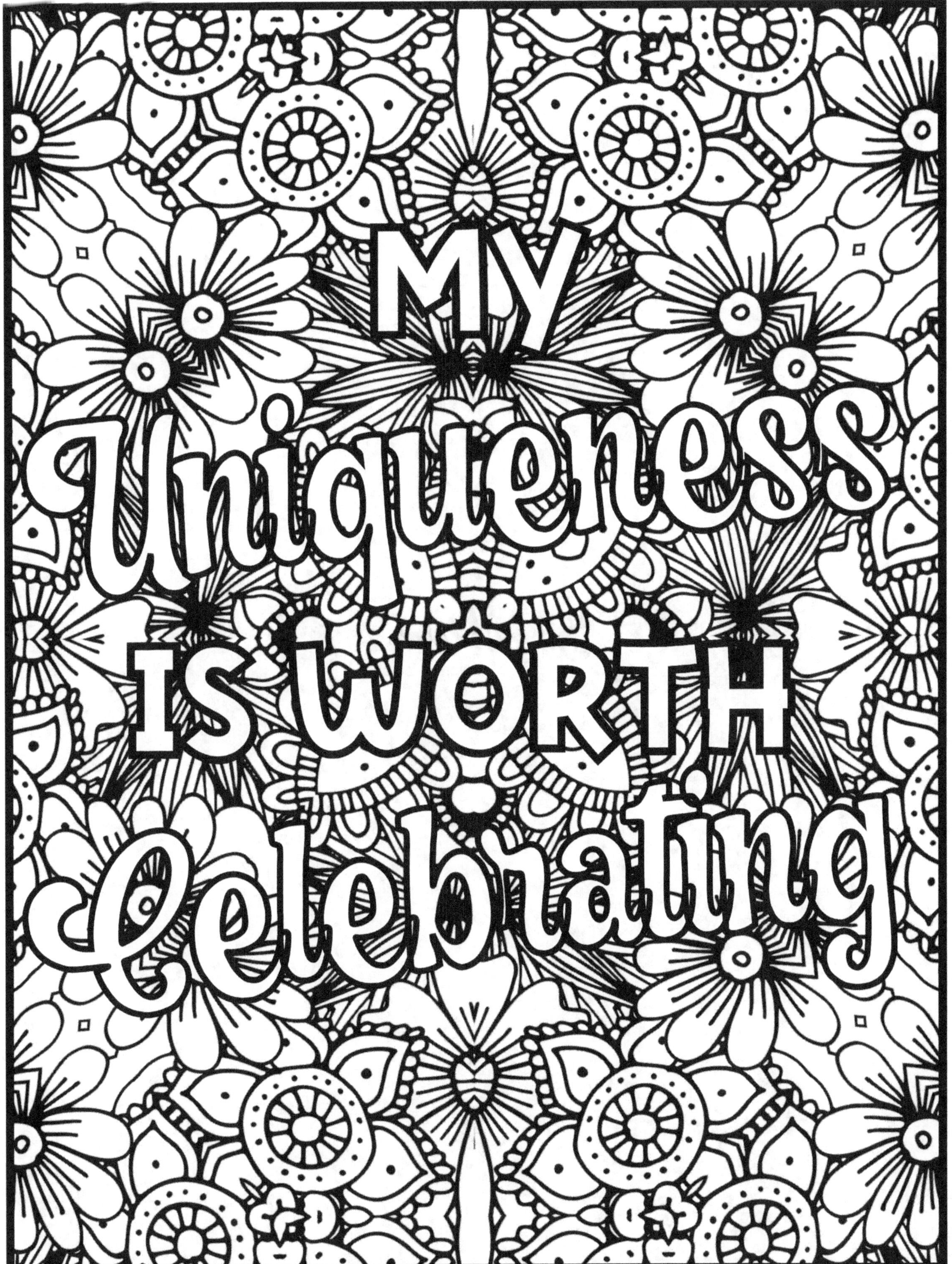

My
Uniqueness
is worth
Celebrating

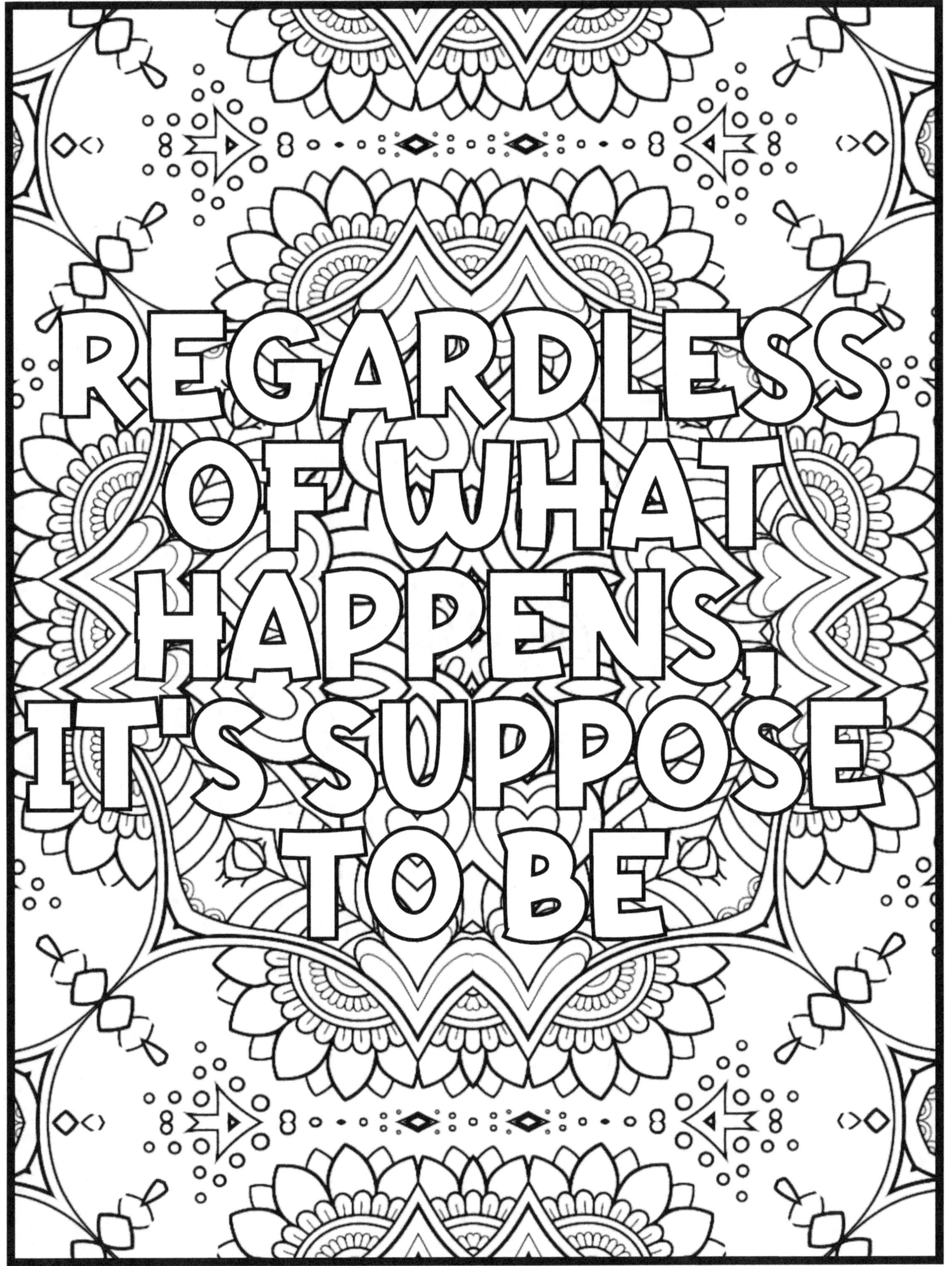

REGARDLESS OF WHAT HAPPENS, IT'S SUPPOSE TO BE

BinkyPetal's
adult coloring books

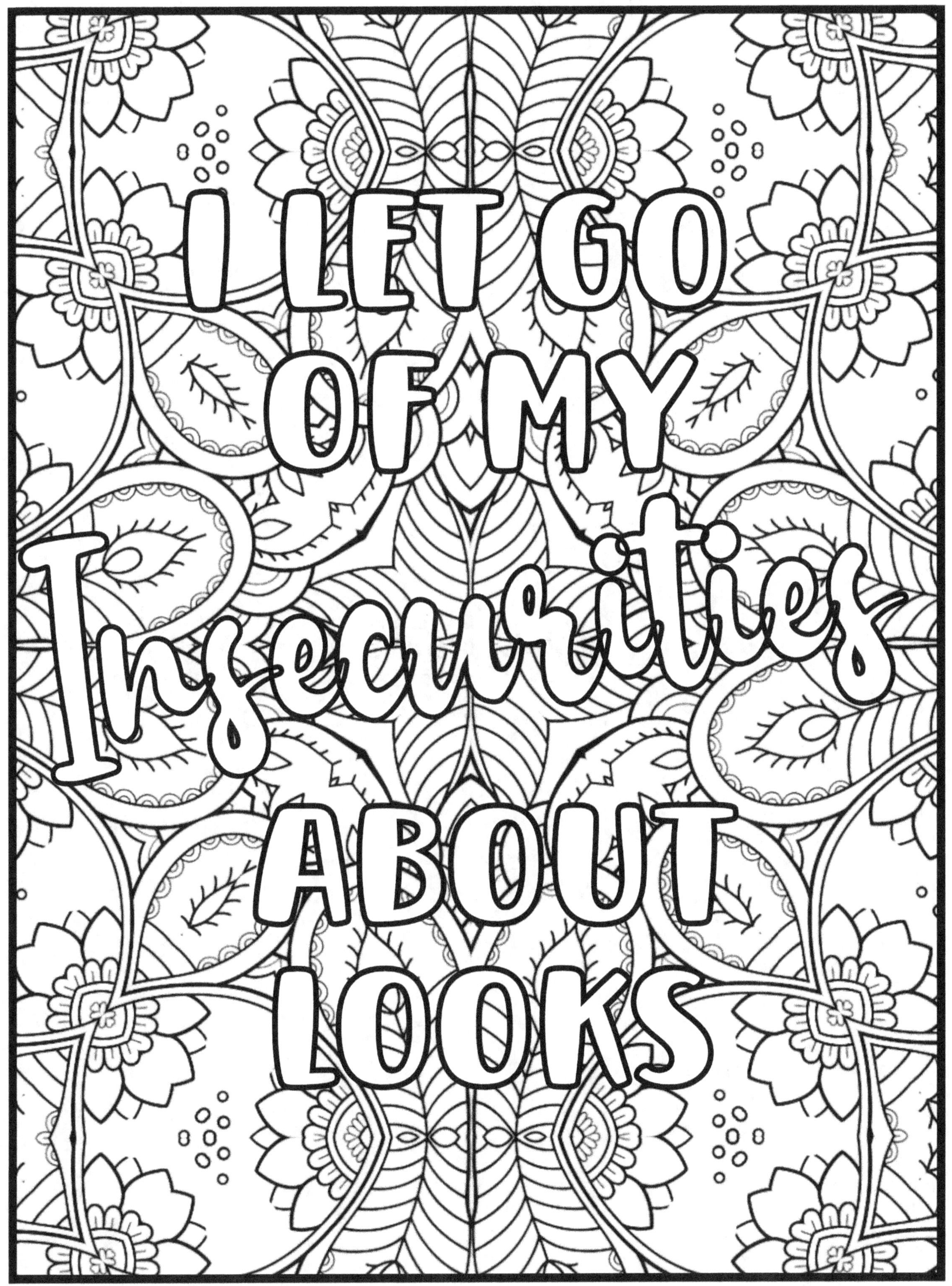
I LET GO
OF MY
Insecurities
ABOUT
LOOKS

BinkyPetal's
adult coloring books

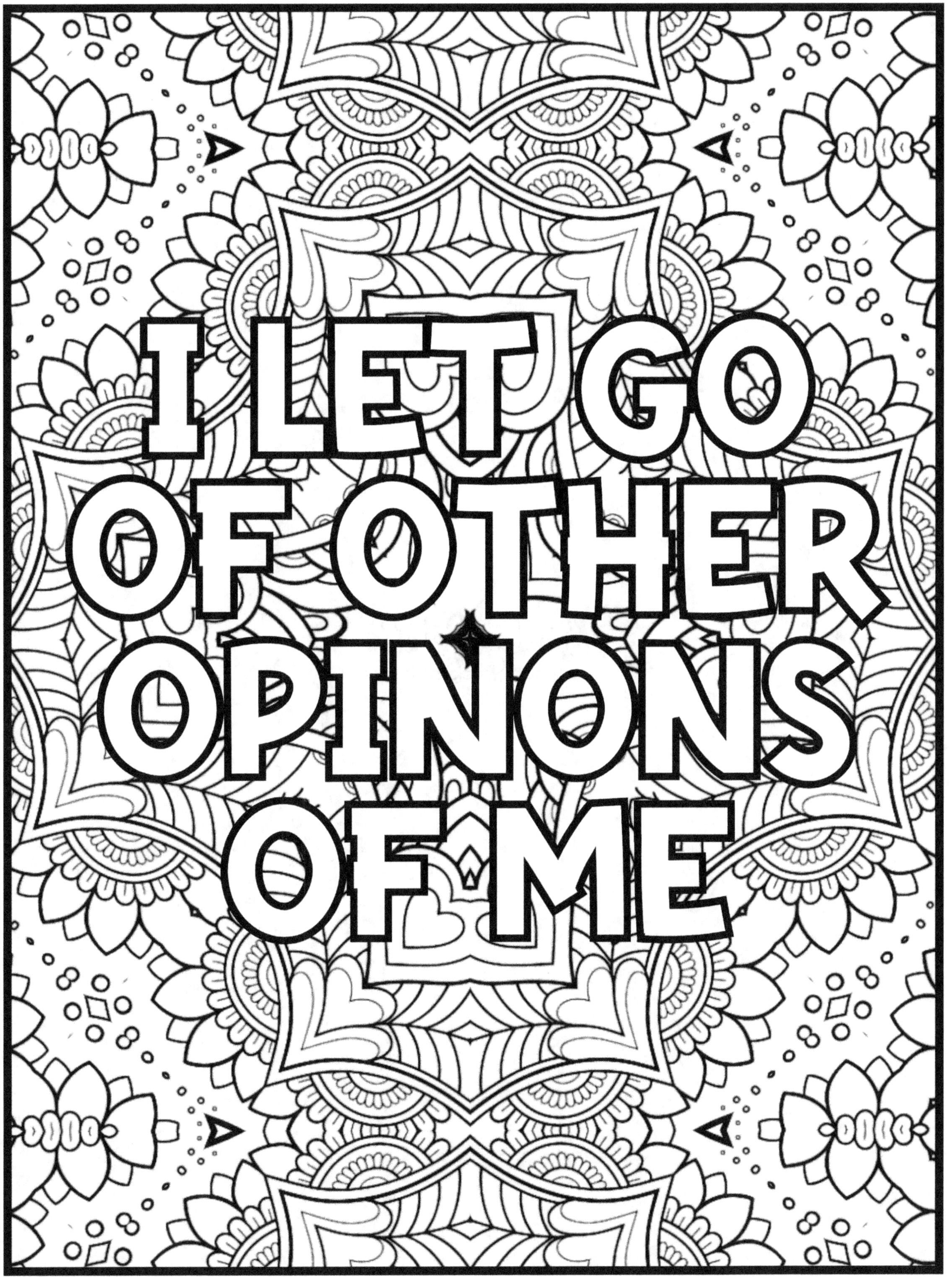

I LET GO
OF OTHER
OPINONS
OF ME

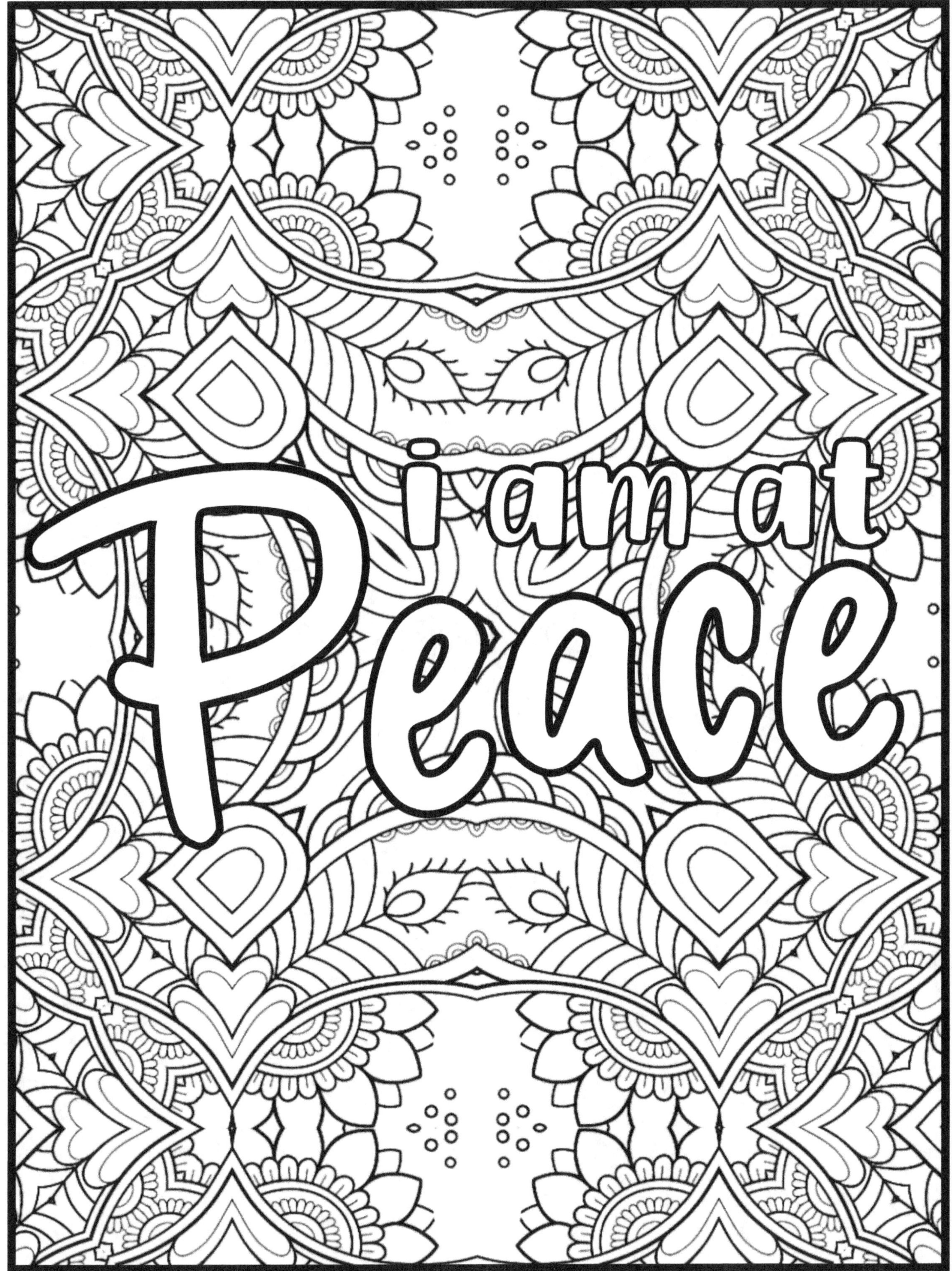

i am at
Peace